barcode on ne[xt page]

D1221470

BST

SPORTS & STRESS THERAPY

Athletic Rehabilitation on
Massage, Stretching & Strengthening

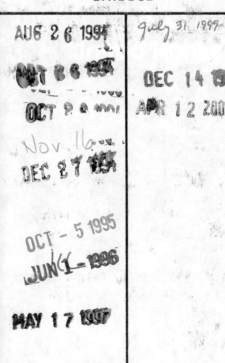

ii

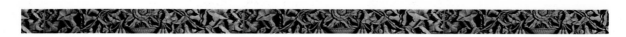

Copyrights

Disclaimer

This book is designed to provide accurate information in regard to the subject matter covered. The responsibility for any adverse effects or consequences from the misapplication of injudicious use of information in this book is the readers. The publisher and author are not engaged in rendering medical or professional service. Readers should use their own judgment or consult their personal physicians for specific applications to their individual problems.

Library of Congress Card Number 93-74515

ISBN 0-9639757-8-1

Production Director: W. K. Tee
Development Editor: Judy LeBlanc
Assistant Editor: Laura Burchett, Dave Henley, Diana Woodard
Project Coordinator: Johari Mohd Said
Proofreader: Geraldine Harding
Text Layout: W. M. Chen, M. S. Heng
Text Design: W. M. Chen
Cover Design: Paul Bagley (Creative Marketing)
Interior Art: Razmah Kassim, Anna Chin
Models: Jarrod Hanks, Stacy Case, Tanya Christie
Photographer: Eddie Edge, Russell Cook
Colour Separation: Aikitar Graphic
Printer: Laser Press Sdn Bhd

Printed in Malaysia

Publisher:
ESKAY INC.
P. O. Box 14266,
Oklahoma City,
Oklahoma, 73113,
USA.
Fax: (405) 721-1016

Malaysia Office:
Rebound Sports Tech Sdn Bhd (MAL)
29, Jalan Bandar Dua,
53100 Kuala Lumpur,
Malaysia.
Tel: (603)-4561208
Fax: (603)-4575835

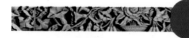
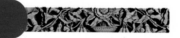

Dedication

This book is dedicated to my wife Raz and son Zakry
who supported me through my
trails and achievements, who has also taught me a new meaning
of life through unconditional love.

Most of all, this book is dedicated to all the athletes
who sacrificed their bodies to endless hours of training and competition.

In loving memory of
Lloyd Keith Price and Dan Kavanaugh.

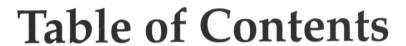

Table of Contents

CHAPTER 5

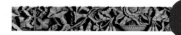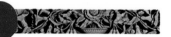

Foreword

Barry Switzer
Former University of Oklahoma Football Head Coach

I first met Eskay four years ago at the University of Oklahoma. I sought him out, because I heard about a young man who had a special gift for helping injured athletes. Since I have been involved in athletics my entire life, a coach the greater part of it, this was something I had to witness personally.

After watching the "Eskay Technique" I was stunned. The methods Eskay used, seemed to be quite simple. My first thought was, why hasn't anyone done this before?

What he is able to do for athletes is nothing short of miraculous. His knowledge of the human body and how it functions while performing is unparalleled.

I spent many hours getting to know Eskay and his philosophy on healing. I am now involved in a physical therapy clinic called "Rebound Oklahoma" and Eskay is a permanent member of our staff. I am privileged to see the results of the "Eskay Technique" on a daily basis and it is truly remarkable. Not only does he possess the ability to help these athletes on a personal level, he also teaches them how to care for themselves. This is the real magic--being able to convey these healing procedures to the athletes themselves. This translates into fewer injuries, quicker rehabilitation time and cost savings since the athletes can perform most of the treatments themselves.

I wish everyone could be as privileged as I have been to see Eskay's work personally, but through this book I honestly feel that the "Eskay Technique" can be passed on to people around the world.

In closing I can only say that Eskay not only has a unique talent but is also one of the kindliest, most sincere, and caring person I have ever met. I am proud he is my friend and associate.

Barry Switzer

Robert D. Lonion, M.D.

*M*edicine in the United States is currently in a state of crisis. Politicians and economists argue that our country's financial existence is directly connected to the increasing cost of medical care. The cost of medical care in the United States is clearly higher than in other parts of the world, yet several million individuals have little access to medical care for lack of medical insurance. This has resulted in a critical examination of the medical profession from a cost benefit point of view as well.

Back injury and back pain represent the most common cause of time lost from work, excluding the common cold. The demand from employers for more effective treatments of back pain and injuries has increased use of MRI scans, surgery, and work hardening programs. Unfortunately, the accompanying cost increase has not been associated with a similar increase in effectiveness. An effective modality or technique for treating, diagnosing, and preventing problems is clearly needed. A program to significantly improve the effectiveness of treatment, even without decreasing the cost, would be significant and a major step forward. However, if an effective modality of treatment were available that would dramatically decrease the cost of the diagnosis, active treatment, and future treatment of these problems, such a technique would be described as miraculous. In my opinion the technique for diagnosis and treatment which have been developed and practiced by Mr. Eskay Shazryl meets those criteria.

I have become acquainted with Eskay and the effectiveness of his therapy through my treatment of patients in primary care medicine. As a Board certified internist who treats a significant number of individuals in sports medicine, rheumatology, and injuries related to occupational medicine, I have received direct feedback from patients whom I referred for physical therapy to Rebound Oklahoma in Oklahoma City. At this facility these individuals received treatment from Eskay and spontaneously praised the effectiveness of his techniques. These individuals had undergone surgery for injuries to the spine or extremities, had tried work hardening programs, and had received treatment such as epidural steroid injections, all without sufficient relief to return to work or sports activities. The "Eskay Technique," when applied effectively, represents what I believe to be the most efficacious and cost effective mode of treating the problems described in this book. The "Eskay Technique" is not designed as an isolated modality of treatment and does not conflict with conventional methods of diagnosis and treatment, physical therapy, manipulation or chiropractic treatment, or specific disciplines such as the McKenzie Technique or the technique of treating myofascial pain and dysfunction as described by Drs. Travell and Simons in their texts. The Eskay Technique significantly decreases the need for invasive treatment while being equally or more effective than the invasive modalities.

Eskay has described the basis of his technique in this book, **Sports and Stress Therapy**. It is well illustrated, not voluminous, but the techniques are extremely effective and powerful when applied appropriately with discipline. The fact that the book can be read easily should not cause the reader to underestimate the effectiveness of the techniques. These techniques are extremely useful and should be integrated in the standard practice of sports medicine, orthopedics, and primary care medicine.

Eskay addresses the treatment of "myofascial trigger points" using the Eskay Technique. I recognize that the very existence of myofascial trigger points is controversial in medical practice, however, the excellent text published by Drs. Travell and Simons and the unquestioned effectiveness of the treatment of these problems has resulted in greater acceptance and objectivity. Based on the effective treatment of several patients whom I have referred to Eskay and the effective treatment of other individuals, including world class Olympic gymnasts, professional hockey players, professional and college football players, and others, Eskay's method of diagnosis and treatment are extremely effective and sometimes superior to conventional physical therapy, surgery, and other modalities.

I strongly encourage the use of the "Eskay Technique" in sports and medical practice for the treatment and prevention of injury and those illnesses which are directly addressed in Eskay's book. The individual who applies his techniques with discipline and common sense will find the Eskay Technique to be an effective treatment and/or prevention of the problems Eskay describes in his book.

Dr. Lonion.

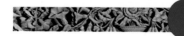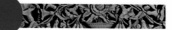

Acknowledgments

*W*ithout the help of thousands of friends, athletes and patients who through the years provided me with valuable information and inspiration in putting together my five years research, this book could not have been written. I wish to recognize and thank them for their contributions:

- YB Haji Abdul Ghani Osman, Malaysian Minister of Youth and Sports, YB Nasruddin Saidin, Dato' Mazlan Ahmad, the Director General of the Malaysian Sports Council and Radzali Hassan who help promote preventive awareness program for athletes in Malaysia.

- Dave Henley, Women Gymnastic Assistant Head Coach at University of Oklahoma, who is a great friend, technical advisor, editor, and a computer genius.

- The Men and Women Head Coach, Greg and Becky Buwick, whom didn't even know that they provided encouragement that helped create this book that serves as a practical guide for all athletes.

- Coach Donny Duncan and Don Jimmerson, The University of Oklahoma Athletic Director and the assistant Athletic Director for their faith and confidence in my capabilities.

- Dr. Sands from University of Utah, who have provided encouragement and assistance in numerous ways and getting my foot into the United States Gymnastic Federation.

- Mr. Larry Derryberry, my most favourite pal, attorney and advisor, who always helps put me back on the right track.

- Dr. Robert Lonion a guru in human body who taught me some of the most important things I've ever learned and gave me tons of important feedback for which I had been searching for years.

- Judy LeBlanc, my great editor for assisting me in the rewriting of the final manuscript. Her superb writing skills, and hard work helps make the book readable.

- I would particularly like to thank both the men and women gymnastic teams at University of Oklahoma for their continued help and support during our research.

- Joan Gilliam, Joy and Chesley Thomas, my foster parents whom I really love and care for.

- Claudia Bullard, my physical therapy consultant, Nick Z. Young, Ross Pebworth, Charles Duke, Mary Jackson, Keri Henderson, Darla Light, Carla Preston and Allen Berryman for the invaluable technical help provided by them at work daily.

- Haji Zulkarnian Hassan, Johari Mohd Said, W.K. Tee, W.M. Chen, M.S. Heng, Ismail Abdul Rahman and Haji Sujaidi Dasuki my Malaysian Counterpart.

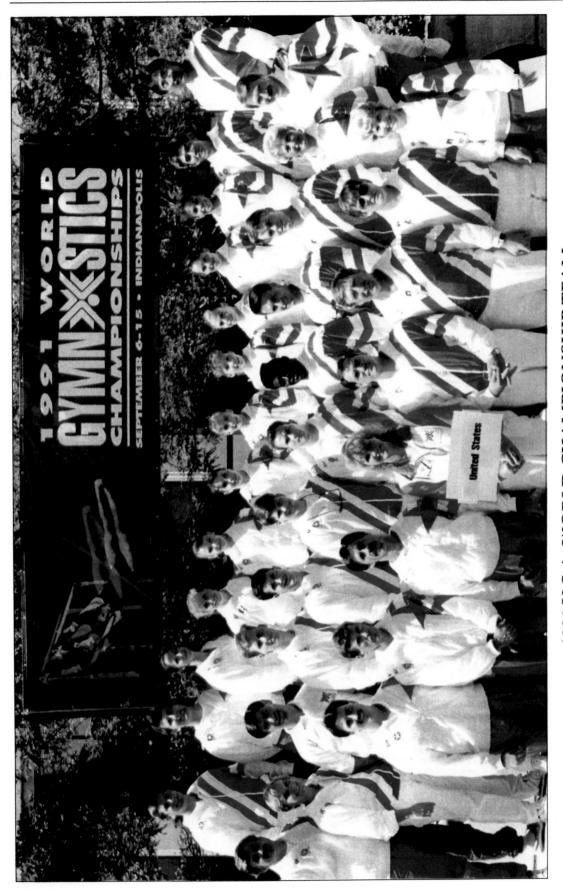

1991 U.S.A. WORLD CHAMPIONSHIP TEAM

Chapter 1

Secrets Of My Success

By Jarrod Hanks

*I*n July of 1990, I was in the gym at the University of Oklahoma training for the McDonald's Challenge: U.S.A. vs. U.S.S.R. Becky Buwick, the University of Oklahoma Women's gymnastics coach, introduced us to our team's newest consultant, Eskay Shazryl.

Eskay watched my workouts and talked about helping me to relieve stress and feeling better, thus performing at my peak. He suggested my training and competition lacked concentration and recuperative technique for relief from intensive training. I never had anyone talk about that before. On the other hand, I was open to suggestions. I was ranked 15th nationally--far short of what I considered my full potential and the Olympic dream.

Eskay proved to be the missing rung on the ladder to the top. Eskay saw an oversight in my training regimen in that there was no recuperative and rehabilitative period for me to recover from a series of rigorous workouts or injuries. Unfortunately, this potentially harmful gap is common in many fitness programs.

The objective of training is to apply physical stress to the body in amounts that can be overcome and compensated for in a short period of time. When successful, the body performs at higher, stronger levels than before, both mentally and physically. If the increased stress becomes extreme, however, either from brief, intense episodes or prolonged exposure, the body fatigues and both mental and physical performances become more difficult. Injuries and "dis-ease" are then more frequent which, in turn, force the athlete to a period of inactivity and rest so the body can restore itself to its original state of good health.

Regardless of the stress encountered, the body reacts and compensates for its effects through changes in bodily functions. The type of stress, its severity and duration, and the initial fitness of the body determine how stress affects the body and how much time is required for compensation and recuperation. This can range from a few minutes to hours, days, months, and longer.

Because of a variety of anatomical differences, some athletes are more prone to injury than others. Loose or tight joints, strength imbalance, muscle weakness, and lopsided training can result in inadequacies in an athlete's level of fitness and stamina. Poor endurance leads to fatigue, slow reaction time, and poor coordination. Stretching and strengthening exercises are essential elements of a sound training program for a safe, healthy athletic performance.

For generations, coaches and researches have identified various methods of training athletes which increase the athletes ability to be more productive and perform at higher levels and reduce the possibility of injury. These have included physiological testing for strength, flexibility and cardiovascular fitness, neuromuscular coordination testing and training, psychological evaluation, relaxation and mental imagery techniques, diet and nutrition programs, development of training cycles, injury rehabilitation therapy, and more.

Each of these methods has proven effective in training athletes with the ideal program combining the best techniques from each area of study. One aspect, however, that is sometimes overlooked when planning the training program, is rehabilitation and recuperation of the athlete from injuries and series of workouts.

While it can be said that if athletes are following a thorough training program, eating properly and getting adequate rest, they are in a recovered state and ready to continue training. Unfortunately, this isn't always the case. Coaches or athletes become overly zealous during training and push for greater performances beyond what is planned in practice. In addition, training, travel, and competition are seldom scheduled with sufficient time allotted for rest and recuperation. There are other variables outside of training that coaches do not consider but which the athlete must contend with and attempt to control. These include school, homework, social pressures, family life, nutritional habits, sleep time, injuries and more. An overabundance of any of these factors could force the individual into a period of reduced activity or even complete rest to allow the body to restore itself into a state of good health. As a result, athletes show inconsistency, perform wearily and at subnormal levels while furthering their risks of injury. This over-fatigued state is called the "Gray Zone." When an athlete is in the Gray Zone, mental and physical performances are difficult and the possibility of injury is enhanced. The combination of continuous training and a rigorous competition schedule triggers fluctuating levels of mental and physiological stress which manifests as wear and tear on the body.

Eskay and I realized I needed a simple, effective stress-relieving technique incorporated into my training to reduce the level of fatigue in the body and thus prevent injuries.

Our goal was to develop a program to permit maximum freedom of movement in every part of the body with minimum effort or stress.

With Eskay's background as an expert in body works technique, athletic injuries and acupuncture and my training regimen as a testing ground, we developed massage techniques which allowed me to unstress and relax quickly after training sessions or competition. Eskay developed the "Foot Method" where athletes walk on each other for 10 or 15 minutes to decrease muscle hypertonicity and to prevent injuries. The Foot Method relaxes the muscles, rejuvenates energy, and enables me to fully stretch out before training. Then all those benefits you get from the Foot Method before a good workout, I get after a good workout too, releasing the stress of training.

After a workout, it can put me to sleep. Believe it or not, I can actually go to sleep with someone walking on my back. It's that relaxing. If I am tense, hurt or in pain, I won't get a good night's sleep. Massage helps me sleep better and that is when I am recuperating--it's an eight-hour process.

Eskay presented the Foot Method to the men's and women's gymnastics teams at the University of Oklahoma and everybody loves it. All we have to say to each other is, "Eskay me". One of the biggest faults athletes have is waiting until after the fact to take care of injuries. By implementing the Eskay Technique religiously, we definitely prevent them.

Eskay's technique helped us overcome objections for not wanting to integrate massage into our daily lives, i.e., conventional or traditional massage is hard to learn, time-consuming, single-minded, and, above all else, extremely tiring for the giver.

The domestication of massage depends on three factors. It must be **simple, efficient** and **effective**. Eskay's technique relies on these three factors and teaches how to promote self-healing by incorporating therapeutic massage into our daily routines with stretching and strengthening exercises for flexibility and stamina.

Eskay also developed what we call "Advance Techniques" which release tight spasms all over the body. Tension in one part of the body causes overexertion and/or compensation in another. A tight thigh muscle will put pressure on the knee. Tightness in the back will put pressure on shoulders and neck. Advance Techniques release the tension and your body relaxes.

After we put Eskay's methods to work for us, the University of Oklahoma gymnastics team realized a 65% decrease in injuries and won the 1991 NCAA Championship. At the same time I was awarded the prestigious NCAA Nissen Award, an honor designating the outstanding male gymnast in collegiate gymnastics. But that wasn't all. I kept winning. In 1991 I qualified for the Pre-Olympic meet in Barcelona, Spain, and the Team U.S.A. World Championships in Indianapolis, Indiana. That same year I finished fifth all-around in the Chunichi Cup competition in Nagoya City, Japan, and I took first in the high bar at the Tokyo Cup. In 1992, I won first all-around at the McDonald's American Cup in Orlando and first all-around at the U.S.A. national championships. I pulled myself up through the national rankings from 15th in 1990 to 7th in 1991 and in 1992, I was number one. It takes more than a good coach, a good club and me to be where I am today. And Eskay made the difference.

And these techniques are curative as well. About two weeks before the American Cup competition, I dislocated my ankle during training. With one week to go, Eskay worked it out and reinlocated (sic) my ankle--the talus bone. I stood up and about 80% of the pain was gone. A week later I won the 1992 American Cup. .

Eskay's techniques are included in my daily physical training. Without help releasing the stress in my body, during long competitions--sometimes as many as four competitions in three days--I wouldn't have been able to go on. Eskay taught me to take care of my body before I tear it up.

I'm 100% sold on Eskay's techniques--so sold, in fact, that I assisted Eskay in presenting the techniques to the recent 51-nation scientific/medical symposium of the International Gymnastics Federation in Indiana. We revealed the findings of the two year comparison study at the University of Oklahoma in the prevention and recuperation of injuries. That distinguished international gathering gave Eskay and his techniques its prestigious endorsement.

Jarrod Hanks

Fitness Transformation

Jarrod's testimonial and his record in the athletic arena speak for themselves. He is proof of the power we possess to control our physical and mental well-being. However, this text is not written solely for Olympic-bound athletes; anyone can benefit from the techniques presented here.

The great performances from teams and individual athletes of the world is the result of many years of planning and training. One country's culture, its population, or its wealth does not provide an advantage or disadvantage in attaining high levels of athletic success. The single, most-important factor in attaining success in athletics is planning for success.

An athlete in motion is a combination of strength, power, speed, grace, and agility. With proper training each of these qualities will develop in harmony with the other. A high performance level is the result of well-planned training sessions and hard work. Developing the proper training regimen requires a well conceived plan--one that develops the unique disciplines in the specific sport in training. No athletes plan to fail, they just fail to plan.

The development of an athletic training agenda involves the same principles of setting goals used in any business success. It begins with well-defined achievement objectives based on a thorough understanding of the sport and its competitors. Then a systematic series of goals and rewards are realized in increasingly difficult stages to accomplish those objectives.

Today's competitors train harder than ever before. They push their minds and bodies through grinding, daily routines that challenge both their mental and physical capacity. Competition is at an all-time high intensity and the performance required to compete at these levels is steadily rising. Yesterday's accomplishments quickly become today's standard. This type of daily challenge results in mental and physical stress that must be compensated and overcome.

When the mind and body are required to perform at unrelenting, escalating levels, stress increases proportionally. If the stress persists, either from continued brief intensive episodes or prolonged exposure beyond the body's immediate or short term recuperative powers, the athlete becomes fatigued. In this fatigued state, referred to as the "Gray Zone," mental and physical performances are inconsistent and decline, and the possibility of injuries increase. This could force the athlete into a period of reduced activities or even complete bed rest to allow the body to restore itself to a state of good health.

Development of a sound prevention and rehabilitation program produces high‑ quality athletes. This book, Sports and Stress Therapy provides a proven technique to help athletes, coaches, trainers, parents, massage and physical therapists combat the fatigue inherent in the Gray Zone and promote peak athletic performance. The techniques emphasize preventive and recuperative methods and, consequently, improve overall performance.

The text covers more than the scope of massage, stretching, and strengthening strategies, however, by explaining the concepts, history and traditions of this technique. In addition, I reveal, through easy to understand explanations and step-by-step illustrations, simple and unique therapy techniques to prevent common acute and/or chronic muscular pains in the neck, shoulder, back, knees, shins, and more. I will show you how massage can revitalize each area and can relieve fatigue after workouts and athletic performance. Next, I will show you how to stretch and strengthen the body after pain reduction therapy which allows the body to perform at its best. I will show you how to balance the mind and body to increase physical energy and to promote a flow of healing energy.

Evolution of the Eskay Techniques

Original ancient Malaysian therapy called "Urut" involved deep tissue massage, using acupuncture points and manipulation of vertebrae, joints, muscles and nerves. The ancient art of healing was preventive and curative, and it is far too complicated for me to put to paper and to explain. It contained many ethnic Malaysian terms which I cannot translate. However, I adapted these terms and some of the complicated movements so that they can be easily understood and mastered.

Eleventh century Malaya was a cultural crossroads of Eastern and Western commerce and traditions. The seaport city of Malacca had a "modern" harbor and was a preferred port of trade providing a halfway point between the Indian Ocean and South China Sea for both European and Oriental sailors. Friendly trade wind blew traders into its sheltered ports to trade goods, to seek spices, to spread religion, and to enhance healing information. Thus, Malacca emerged a prosperous, influential frontier—a veritable melting pot of commerce, religion and medicine.

Malacca became an important "information exchange center" for healers, such as "Bomoh" (Malaysian medicine men who served as both religious healers and psychic), Buddhist monks, Chinese acupuncturists, Ayurvedic medicine men (from East India), and others who exchanged their unique concepts of religion, culture and medicine. The most beneficial contributions to Malaysian traditional medicine were: Chinese acupuncture, herbal and aroma therapy (incense), martial arts, Taoism and Buddhism; East Indian Ayurvedic medicine, massage, meditation, Hinduism; Middle Eastern Islamic religious healing approach, Islam; and Western Christianity and European healing dimensions and ideologies.

Each contributing culture produced enterprising gurus, each possessing such fervor in their beliefs that local interest in other worlds spread. Malaysia's cosmopolitan tradition, strategic location, and international exposure enlightened Malaysian "touch healers" to new approaches and ideologies. As a result of mass cultural fusion, these holistic methods integrate the disciplines and traditions of diverse countries. Through curiosity and integration of cross-cultural information, Malaysian tradition became unique, blending the best of new information with traditional know how into a technique called "Urut."

Bomohs shared their healing heritage and martial arts with their descendants. "Bidan", Malaysian midwives, taught female family members special herbal remedies, massage moves and natural delivery techniques; Buddhist monks and priests preserved secret developments and improvised "foreign" techniques within temple walls.

Eventually, however, modern medicine and miracle quick-fix drugs created a cultural shift from traditional medicine as a single form of healing. Unfortunately, traditional touch healing and ancient disciplines have almost vanished from contemporary Malaysian culture, surviving mainly in remote villages and temples.

The idea of producing a high-quality prevention and rehabilitation program has been in development for several years. I spent years researching injuries with Malaysian healers, acupuncturist, medical doctors, chiropractors, sports trainers, physical therapists and athletes. I combined several cultural and therapeutic disciplines and medical know-how into this unique massage system that I call "The Eskay Technique."

The Eskay Technique involves only **muscle** and **"Trigger Point"** manipulation and is useful as both preventive and curative disciplines. Learning these vital skills and techniques enable anyone to experience the phenomenon of natural self-healing.

The first method to understand is the Basic Technique—Foot Method, which was initially developed to alleviate the effects of fatigue and speed up the recovery process of injured athletes at the University of Oklahoma. The Foot Method is a pressure/compression technique which relieves muscular tension from the back, arms, hips, and legs by using one or two feet to make rocking and/or stepping motions over the body. It is easy to learn and takes less than 20 minutes to perform. The Foot Method massage technique makes daily massage sessions possible for every athlete, parent and coach.

The Advance Techniques are based on a lifetime of study of touch therapy and incorporate many of the Malaysian healing arts. These techniques introduce a precise approach for specific problems in every part of the body. As you prepare to use the Advance Techniques, you will learn how to develop and to utilize the strength in your **hands, elbows, feet,** and **body weight** as your set of massage "tools". These "tools" are then used to apply the **Kneading Technique** for general relaxation, the **Scorpion Technique** for precise kneading action, the **Thumb Technique** for deeper pressure to precise muscle areas, and **Elbow-Knuckle Technique** for deep muscle friction, and finally, the **Palm Technique** for broad coverage of sensitive areas.

The Advance Techniques involve precise, deep tissue massage on "Trigger Points" to each specific body area. A trigger point is described as the focal point of a muscle in spasm that when pressed, causes pain in other areas of the body. "Trigger Point manipulation" has proved beneficial to athletes who demonstrate a loss of function due to an adaptive shortening of the muscle or adhesions in any soft tissues associated with movement. While mastering these techniques, you will learn the basic anatomy of the neck, back, arms, hips, legs, feet and more. You will learn to recognize the common athletic ailments in specific parts of the body and which massage techniques to use for tension release. Then you will learn to stretch and strengthen each part of your body after pain reduction therapy which allows the body to perform at its best. The ultimate goal is to maximize the body's flexibility and mobility.

Unlike other disciplines which demand strict adherence to the sequence of manipulations or which discourage integration with other therapies, Eskay Techniques are shown for reference, but it is not necessary to perform all of the techniques in sequence for healthful benefits. This is not an all-or-nothing program.

How you benefit from **Sports and Stress Therapy** depends on you. Success relies on your dedication, motivation and drive. I cannot overstate the importance of education and planning when developing a sports program. Great achievements in sports performances cannot be developed overnight; however, great strides can be made in a very short period of time.

Good Luck

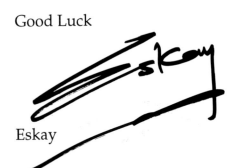

Eskay

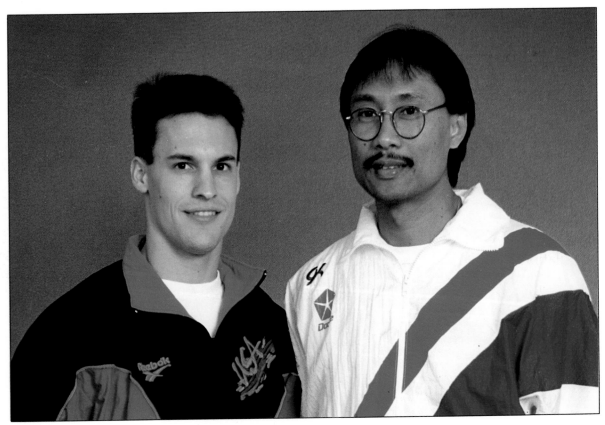

JARROD HANKS & ESKAY SHAZRYL

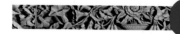 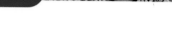

Chapter 2

Body Awareness

"If it's not broken, don't fix it."

This popular old saying has been accepted gospel for generations and it has been applied to everything in our lives from automobile service to our personal health. Yet, ironically, when applied to something as vital as health care, the "if it's not broken" syndrome promotes a backward consciousness that undermines our attempts in a negative, futile way to achieve vigorous wellness and a competitive advantage.

Modern medical science has been highly successful in treating and diagnosing disease, but it has been lax, to say the least, in promoting good health. Health care practitioners are largely obsessed with disease and illness "after the fact," and, like wooden soldiers, we fall in line with them into a dangerous pattern of "treatment" emphasis rather than "prevention" emphasis. Instead of actively participating and planning a strategic, preventive personal health care plan while we are healthy, we participate only when illness or injury dictates that we do. This attitude is detrimental in preventing future problems and, in the end, it is disruptive, costly, and sometimes fatal.

When we think about preventive health care programs, vitamin supplements, inoculations and immunizations come to mind. While these are essential components of longevity, they remain only a minor part of overall prevention. A fitness life-style that includes a balanced and nutritious diet, an optimistic attitude, adequate sleep and rest, regular exercise, and stress management is paramount to preventing injury and illness. In order to take responsibility for our own good health, we need to understand exactly what optimal health—or wellness—means. The absence of illness does not necessarily imply good health. Good health can be present to some degree, but not to its full potential.

To achieve optimal health, above all else, we must heighten our sense of awareness of our body's function. And to benefit fully from this awareness, we must understand natural body processes. When we are unable to see, feel or hear subtle body signals that reveal early telltale signs of internal dysfunction, we are strangers to our own bodies and risk all hope for healthy longevity. It isn't necessary, however, to bombard ourselves with extensive, technical medical data. Unfortunately, many of us know more about our car engines than we do about the internal mechanics of our bodies.

When we learn to rely on awareness, we are able to recognize subtle, yet potentially harmful, health conditions. When we are in fine tune with our bodies, we easily recognize the little symptoms that tell us we are out of sync and we can quickly and effortlessly remedy detrimental conditions. Early detection of simple, minor symptoms is the first step in creating awareness and developing a personalized preventive health care and fitness plan.

Unfortunately, we are an impatient society which tends to seek instant gratification and immediate, visible results from our efforts, and perfect health won't happen overnight. We can hardly place the blame on the heads of ignorant physicians. Most health practitioners realize that if they told us to change our eating habits, join an aerobics class, meditate, treat ourselves to a professional massage, and sleep more, rest more, play more and pray more, we would walk right out of the office and get a second opinion. It is far easier for them to reach for the prescription pad than to convince us we are the victim of our own failure. Like anything worthwhile, good health takes time and results are far reaching yet subtle externally and invisible internally. In a fairly short time, however, it is possible to prevent current problems from worsening and developing into potentially dangerous health concerns that leave us on the sideline. In our enthusiasm to achieve too much too fast, we often defeat ourselves in the process and find ourselves with time on our hands waiting for an injury to heal.

Medical advances have improved quality of life and, in many cases, saved countless lives. Disease control and medical breakthroughs have provided us with useful information about ways to live healthier, longer lives. While medical science has taken giant strides since the days of bloodletting and "hack" surgery, the basic source of disease has not changed since then—we have merely found "academic explanations" for it. Even in prehistoric times, **"STRESS"** was a killer. And although we don't have to live under the threats of freezing winters or attacking woolly mammoths, we live in a demanding, hostile world none the less. While medicine cures symptoms, we are still searching for ways to find permanent solutions to the ravages of demands we put on ourselves. Doctors alleviate the symptoms and dull our pains, we ultimately begin a cycle of temporary solutions, patching and mending the fabric of our culture. We fail to address the life-threatening elements that contribute to the onset of disease and illness—tension, **STRESS** and fatigue.

The Power of Touch

Touch is nature's therapy; it introduces natural abilities enhancing health and lifestyle. Everyone is born with a natural instinct to touch and be touched and we have long recognized the human hand as a powerful tool possessed with healing properties.

Touching, especially through massage, creates healing potential, transferring energy which soothes, heals and relays feelings of sharing and nurturing. Touching enables the surrounding world to be "sensed".

Our sense of touch depends upon the functions of the skin, the largest organ of the body. Our skin is unevenly covered with sensitive nerve endings. With high sensitivity areas, such as the fingertips, and low sensitive areas, such as the back, these nerve endings act as sense receptors. All of our senses—sight, taste, hearing, smell and touch—rely on nerve endings. When touch is sensed, such as heat, cold, pressure and pain, cutaneous nerve endings are at work.

The various receptors within the skin and body perform specific tasks. Free nerve endings found everywhere in the skin respond slowly to touch and pressure. These receptors react to the slightest brush of the skin or even before the skin is touched. Deeper nerve endings respond to heavy, continuous pressure changes and vibrations. Nerve endings give dimension to the world we perceive around us. Through a series of intricate nerve impulses or synapses, we use touch to define our reality.

Sense receptors start a chain reaction that enables the brain to instruct the body's internal pharmacy to produce chemicals to control or heal the body. Neurochemical which enable us to feel, to sense, and to emote are synthesized; hormones affecting every organ in our bodies are stimulated by the simple act of touching. These chemical changes help us react to stimuli. When we are stimulated through touch, the brain receives a message via sense receptors that is received, decoded, analyzed and acted upon. Touch calls out and the brain answers—"Ouch!" "It's hot!" "It hurts!" "It feels good!"

Unfortunately, although our sense of touch imparts these therapeutic qualities, we are touching less than ever before. "Socially acceptable" rules of behavior have undermined the instinctive need to touch and to be touched. Mixed messages have been sent to our culture and we are ambivalent about appropriate touch behavior outside our closest intimate relationships. Touching in a business situation is discouraged due in part to a recent flurry of sexual harassment allegations. Children are taught "don't touch" rules which desensitize their natural curiosity. Even close family members are reluctant to touch each other in light of new revelations of the incidence of incest.

Non-touching tendencies have seeped into touching professions as well. Even medical doctors, while recognizing the need for touch is essential for health and survival, sometimes fail to use their own best medical tool—their hands. However, while many traditional physicians balk at using ancient hand on practices, there is a growing legion of doctors who realize the potential of combining modern science with old-fashioned traditions we used to call "bedside manner." These doctors recognize the potential of the hands as a healing tool. By blending natural remedies with modern science, they achieve amazing results.

Why Massage ?

A wise man realizes that there is no single thing better than another. A touch master once said, "Cut a cabbage into four equal parts and give one each to a China man, an Indian, an Englishman and a Malaysian. Ask them to prepare a dish for a feast the following day. You can bet they will all bring a different cabbage dish for the feast, but they all boil down to the same ingredient—cabbage."

Likewise, most massage disciplines have similar purposes but differ in their approaches. The single, primary goal of these techniques is to ease muscle tension and dispel fatigue, which in turn restores normal function to the muscular, nervous, lymphatic and blood circulatory systems. Massage, if done properly, eliminates the underlying causes and sources of pain.

Any type of massage will ultimately be beneficial if done properly. Swedish Massage, Rolfing, Acupressure, Shiatsu, Reflexology, and other methods share similar goals—to use natural healing methods to achieve vital, pain-free health. These disciplines require basic knowledge of human anatomy and physiology.

The Eskay Techniques preserve the basic concept by initiating natural healing. They provide a drug-free, home prevention kit designed to ease aches and pains and to insure continued wellness. It should be understood, however, that to fully benefit from the Eskay Techniques requires practice, discipline and change. We are not born with an inherent map that tracks a journey toward good health. Without academic instructions, it is necessary to utilize all available information. But when we learn to recognize body signals as intelligent "detours" around harmful habits, we are able to compensate for inherent weaknesses within our bodies and to recognize when the body is self-healing.

The Eskay Techniques are able to recondition damaged muscles through deep massage. Exercise bolsters the immune system by stimulating the heart, blood and lymphatic circulation. Exercise, however healthy, causes stress and soreness to the musculatory system, massage eliminates or eases the by products of exercise, such as the accumulation of lactic and uric acid in the muscles.

Over-exertion strains muscle tissue, damages ligaments, tendons and cartilage, produces muscle spasm, creates fibrosis (chronic inflammation caused by binding of muscle tissue), and causes a build-up of waste that leaves muscles stiff. Massage improves blood circulation by encouraging the exchange of oxygenated blood for carbon dioxide wastes, accelerating the flow of blood to the capillaries, veins and arteries.

The lymphatic system plays a dual role, purifying and draining body waste. Lymph is a clear, viscous fluid which is produced in small glands throughout the body. These glands build and transmit white corpuscles into the bloodstream which carry out waste products that accumulate in the muscles. This waste product filters through the kidneys is eliminated by excretion. Since lymph is circulated by the pull of gravity, osmosis, or muscular contraction, manual manipulations provide a little "push," forcing waste products to enter the bloodstream more quickly.

Muscle pain is relieved by improving circulation and lymphatic flow and by breaking up fibrosis that binds muscles together. Fibrosis can also be caused by lack of glycogen and the accumulation of waste products to the muscle fiber. Fibrosis shortens the muscle and produces spasms. Muscle fibers bind together and are unable to function independently and with full mobility. These shortened muscles are easily pulled and torn, and the slow process of micro-trauma creates scar tissue between fibers.

Muscle spasm is a protective, defensive function which makes muscles feel knotted, lumpy or swollen, creating discomfort when fatigued muscle fibers tangle and contract. Muscle soreness is a subtle body signal that tells us, "Stop! You are hurting me." Massage corrects these problems by improving blood circulation, loosening muscle fibers, lengthening muscles, and untying muscle knots. Swelling, soreness and muscle tension is relieved, future injuries are prevented and recovery time is shortened with massage.

Although results are subtle, they are physically and mentally real. By using deep muscle therapy on a regular basis, chronic muscle spasm caused by daily stress is alleviated.

Stretching and Strengthening

A proper warm-up followed by stretching exercises is essential to prevent injury and to enhance performance. Ideally, the body's temperature should elevate 2 degrees Fahrenheit during the warm-up period by jogging, bicycling, walking, or calisthenics. When sweat beads form on the forehead, the body temperature has usually been raised.

Next, each muscle group should be held in a static or passive stretch for 10 to 60 seconds, allowing the muscles to lengthen slowly. Bouncing or "ballistic" stretching will be counterproductive because muscles will reflexively contract when suddenly stretched. Stretching is pleasant and pain free and you should begin to be aware of the muscles' subtle tension, contraction, and relaxation. Stretching lengthens muscles and tendons and makes them pliable. Joint mobility, flexibility and range-of-motion are enhanced and the risk of sprain or strain is reduced.

In addition to stretching exercises, strengthening exercises should be added to training programs for an appropriate balance between flexibility and strength. Strength is the ability of the athlete to do work against resistance or the maximum force or tension the athlete can generate in a single effort.

If resistance is applied to a muscle, it contracts and tears slightly. These "micro-tears" heal slightly shorter and the muscle increases in size and strength. In strength training cycles the muscle is worked to capacity and then the workload is increased. Strength increases stability of joints and enables the athlete to move faster without injury.

Stretching and strengthening exercises must be done together to prevent being what is called "muscle bound." Whenever muscles are strengthened, they must be stretched as well. If flexibility training is not included in strength training, joint mobility and athletic agility decreases.

Soft Tissue Injury

Symptoms such as tight, tender muscles, deep aches and pains and lack of joint mobility are warning signs that the body has suffered soft tissue injury. Soft tissue, which includes muscles, tendons and ligaments, can be damaged by misuse, overuse, lack of use, poor posture or nutrition. Sometimes the damaged tissue heals incorrectly, leaving muscle fibers twisted or knotted. These tender points are called by many different health professionals by many different names, including acupressure points, Ah Shi points, myofasciitis, myofibrositis, fibromyalgia, contraction points, muscle shield, myofascial trigger point and more. Instead of creating another name for almost the same condition, I will rely on the most common descriptive term "Trigger Points." These points often cause pain and limited mobility, especially in the soft tissue of leg, arm, neck, lower back, wrist and even jaw.

The cycle of misuse, damage and pain create a chronic muscle condition called Myofascial Pain Syndrome. Although common, the chronic pain of trigger points are often misdiagnosed, ignored or overlooked. Because of the complexity of the condition and because chronic pain (pain which there doesn't seem to be a cause or physically visible) is often so hard to diagnose, many people go untreated. This type of chronic pain cannot be explained through mechanical tests such as X-rays, MRI's or CAT Scans. The pain is often thought to be psychogenic or "all in the head". It is easy to see how a misdiagnosed trigger point problem could cause distress. Similarly, undiagnosed shoulder, head, and lower back pain are significant causes of lost time and money.

It is important to be able to distinguish between normal, healthy soft tissue and injured tissue. Each muscle is embedded in a layer of fascia, which separates one muscle from another muscle. Normal fascia is soft and pliable, allowing the muscle to contract and lengthen efficiently. When injured, muscles that naturally function separately will form adhesions and will impair the muscles ability to move freely above one another. This causes muscle bonding which restricts flexibility. Healthy tissue does not have tight bands of muscles and fascia; it is free of trigger points or knots. Muscles afflicted with trigger point pain , however, have tight cords of muscle fibers and are generally tender to the touch and refer pain.

Referred pain is another complexity of trigger point pain and another example of how soft tissue problem can be misdiagnosed. Any muscle can develop trigger points and many muscles develop multiple trigger points. Resulting pain, however, is rarely at the spot of the problem—it is referred. Referred discomfort from trigger points usually manifests in deep, dull aches and pains and can vary in intensity from mild to intolerable.

Muscles are abused in many common and complex ways. Muscle cramps, an involuntary muscle contraction, are common athletic complaints caused by biomechanical problems such as bone misalignment or nutrition problems such as mineral deficiencies.

Muscle pulls, similar to muscle cramps, occur when muscle fibers are stretched or contracted involuntarily or beyond their normal limits. Strains and tears occur most often with this kind of forcible resistance.

Direct trauma, probably the most serious abuse to muscle fibers, results from a direct blow, forced motions or rotations, tearing, pulling, and stretching. The immediate effects of trauma to muscle and muscle fibers is a cycle of blood constriction and congestion. After injury blood vessels constrict and inhibit circulation to the damaged area. This constriction starves the injury site of oxygen and nutrients but at the same time allows white blood cells to move toward the injured site. This migration of leukocytes (white blood cells) is called diapedesis.

Diapedesis produces exudate, a fluid rich in protein and antibodies, leaked from blood vessels. This leakage produces swelling, or edema, and often causes inflammation. Inflammation can be recognized by its redness, swelling, local heat, pain and loss of function.

An untreated muscle injury begins a cycle of poor healing and pain. A muscle that heals incorrectly, develops scar tissue, and limits normal muscle movement is a common cause of muscle reinjury and further debilitation. Tiny tears or micro-trauma in the soft tissue then heal but cause underlying muscle fibers to contract, twist and knot. New tissue covers old and fibers tighten creating a lumpy area—the trigger point area. This new tissue is less elastic than the original tissue and causes muscles to shorten, thus decreasing mobility. If injuries are not treated properly, they become chronic and form an immobile scar that permanently reduces the body's range of motion.

Typical injury/trigger point pain cycle can be traced through a series of events. Trauma to muscle leads to involuntary contractions; lead to muscle spasm; muscle spasm leads to trigger points, i.e. Myofascial Pain Syndrome.

If recognized early, minor tissue damage can often be treated successfully and with minimal inconvenience or disability. Improper care of injuries, however, makes the situation worse by delaying healing. Untreated or even worse, mistreated injuries lead to unsightly scarring, permanent disability, and even death. Treatments vary and can include passive and/or, aggressive therapy to repair damage, alleviate pain, diminish symptoms, and prevent injuries from recurring.

Passive treatment of trigger points includes the use of moist heat, ice and rest. Moist heat applied to the chronic injury significantly reduces muscle soreness. Ice therapy requires careful administration since damp, cold weather or chilled muscles can augment chronic, prolonged trigger point pain. But if applied carefully, ice treatment helps reduce inflammation on new or reoccurring acute injuries. Resting an area prevents aggravation or additional trauma to an injury and allows for recuperation.

Active trigger point therapy includes movement, stretching and myofascial release or deep tissue massage. As soon as inflammation subsides, gentle movements encourage natural healing to soft tissue and a subsequent reduction of pain. Stretching improves muscle flexibility and mobility due to hypertonicity thus returning the skeleton to proper biomechanical alignment. Then strengthening allows the athlete to return to play.

The ideal program is progressive with increased performance achieved at each workout until full mobility, balance, coordination, strength, and flexibility are restored. An athlete who returns to competition or full training too early risks additional injury.

However, the most effective active trigger point therapy is deep myofascial release massage. This deep massage increases blood circulation and lengthens the glidability of the muscle fibers. Deep massage on muscles maintains the muscle tissue in the ideal state of nutrition, flexibility, and vitality so that after recovery from trauma or disease, the muscle functions at its maximum. A fatigued muscle is unable to purge itself of toxins. With massage, blood circulation is improved, removal of wastes and toxins from tissues is accelerated, metabolic and oxygenation processes are activated, and the central and peripheral nervous systems' activity is normalized.

In summary, hands heal--not magically, but with systematic finger and body movements that produce equilibrium and holistic results. When body and mind are balanced, a natural state encourages self-healing. But nothing about deep massage is unnatural--just forgotten.

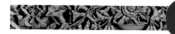

Chapter 3

Eskay Technique
Basic Technique
Foot Method

*T*he Eskay Technique covers more than the basics of ancient massage and includes a complete preventive approach to good health. While preparing the Eskay Technique, I provided for both athletes and non-athletes. Through years of experimentation and observation, I discovered new ways through touch therapy to alleviate the aches and pains associated with daily lifestyle problems and patterns.

I utilized the Eskay Technique on a variety of subjects including paralyzed stroke victims, terminal cancer patients, athletes, medical doctors, chiropractors, massage and physical therapists, and vital, healthy men and women to create viable, beneficial techniques. Subject feedback and analysis showed me the remarkable potential of simple touch therapy. I discovered the need of many people for a quick, effective touch program and I created "The Foot Method."

Initially, The Foot Method was designed specifically for athletes and coaches to address the common, chronic ailments associated with training and competition. This simple, yet effective, technique relieves muscular tension and fatigue. It provides dual benefit by helping to prevent injuries yet bringing the body to an optimum level of relaxation for restoration to occur. The Foot Method is a maintenance technique which brings about immediate, complete relief from physiological and psychological stress.

This preventive massage technique uses a "buddy system" whereby coaches and/or athletes massage each other. After a brief demonstration and practice, the athletes are able to apply the actual manipulations with confidence and without professional supervision. The ease of the massage technique makes daily massage sessions possible for every athlete.

To test the benefits of Eskay Technique-Foot Method, a two-year comparison study of injuries was performed on collegiate female gymnasts at the University of Oklahoma.

During the second year of the study, the Eskay Technique-Foot Method massage was taught and performed daily.

The study revealed that when a balanced combination of skill training, strength and aerobic/anaerobic conditioning, and massage therapy for restoration were used, a 65% reduction in injuries occurred. The study concluded that the Eskay Technique played an important part in reducing levels of fatigue and muscular tension associated with training—a major component in the reduction of injuries.

Through work with gymnasts, wrestlers, runners, football, basketball, and tennis players from the University of Oklahoma, the Foot Method was refined. Its immediate goal was to relieve stress, thus stimulating the recuperative system. When athletes recover quickly, they escape chronic pain and recover more completely. This preventive touch therapy helped the athletes physically and the accompanying relaxation enhanced other aspects of the training process such as sleep, concentration, and competition.

And the benefits continued. By incorporating the "buddy system" into the Foot Method massage, frequent or daily use of the program, when performed properly by these massage amateurs, in this case athletes, created the same benefits—relaxation and tension relief—customarily experienced only from a professional full-body massage.

The specific study on athletes at the University of Oklahoma led me to introduce similar programs to universities nationally. Through reduction of muscle tension and enhanced concentrative skills, athletes who had previously spent painful, sleepless nights following training experienced quality rest that enabled them to train more effectively and that improved their mental clarity in the classroom.

Now, in response to demand from the health community at large, the Foot Method body-works has been adapted to meet the needs of non-athletes as well to enhance physical performance and reduce pain through a combination of relaxation and body manipulations. The techniques outlined here have been simplified and redirected to insure effectiveness and to help alleviate physiological problems before they become acute. Results range from simple stress reduction to pain-free longevity.

The Foot Method is a pressure/compression technique which relieves muscle tension by using one or two feet to make rocking/stepping motions over the body. With the aid of a support chair for added control, it relieves pressure and tension from the receiver's back, hips, thighs, lower legs, arms and feet. This may be the only way to have someone "walk all over you" and feel good about it. Basic techniques, however, must precede advanced techniques and all must be performed frequently or daily to ensure program success.

The Foot Method can be learned and administered in a short time, and it can produce maximum therapeutic results. But, practice, commitment, discipline and personal dedication are essential to success. The technique is part of a preventive mini-massage program which cannot immediately repair years of damage and chronic muscle spasm, but it can aid in the elimination of daily stress, thereby reducing the probability of future injury and pain through enhanced muscle control.

This 20-minute massage program produces rare effects--immediate and maximum relaxation. Excluding chemical treatments and drug therapy, this is one of the few strategies which can produce immediate, soothing, therapeutic effects with minimum effort. In short, the Mini-Eskay Technique is a definite "Stress Buster."

It is important to remember, however, that the Eskay Technique-Foot Method is preventive therapy. If injury indicates curative measures, however, Basic and Advanced-Eskay Technique can coexist with conventional medical treatments for rapid recovery to prevent recurring injury or relapse.

Each of us was born with the innate ability to heal through touch; mastery of this technique brings about maximum stress relief and an improved quality of life. I remember an analogy my Master often used. He said, "Our lives are like a piece of wood and we have two choices. We can preserve and polish the wood, so that it can be handed down for generations; or we can throw it in the river, where it will drift and rot."

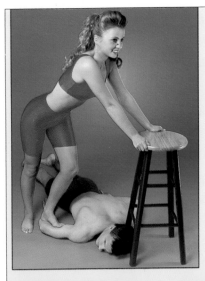

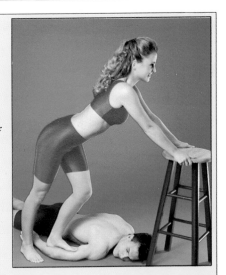

- Have the Receiver lie on his/her stomach.
- Place your support chair on one side of the Receiver and stand on the other side.
- Giver stand on his most stable foot.
- Apply between 70 to 100 pounds of pressure.

Apply technique to both of the Receiver's arms.

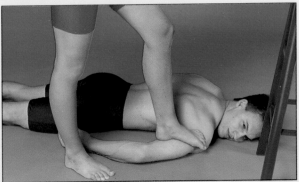

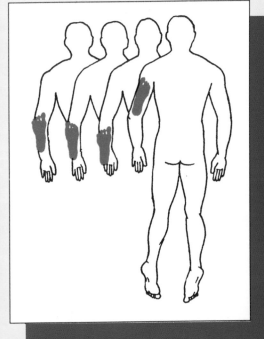

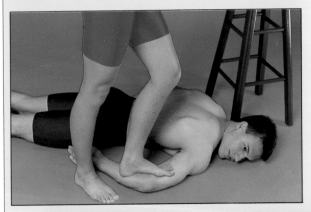

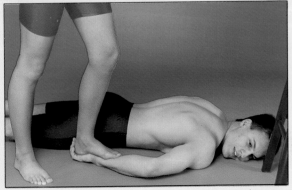

On each step, rest your foot on the Receiver's arm for about 20 seconds. Rock back on to your support foot and then step onto the arm with the other foot. Each time you rock back and alternate feet, move the manipulating foot a little further down the arm. You raise, press, raise, press with rhythmic movement.

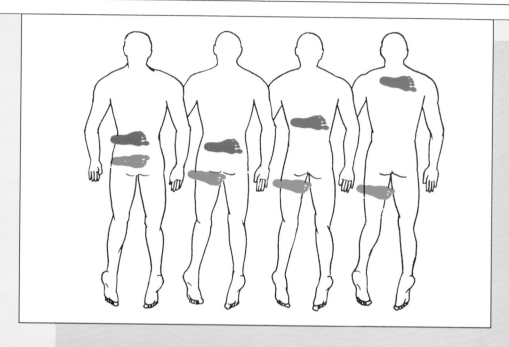

Repeat the process up and down the Receiver's back and both thighs.

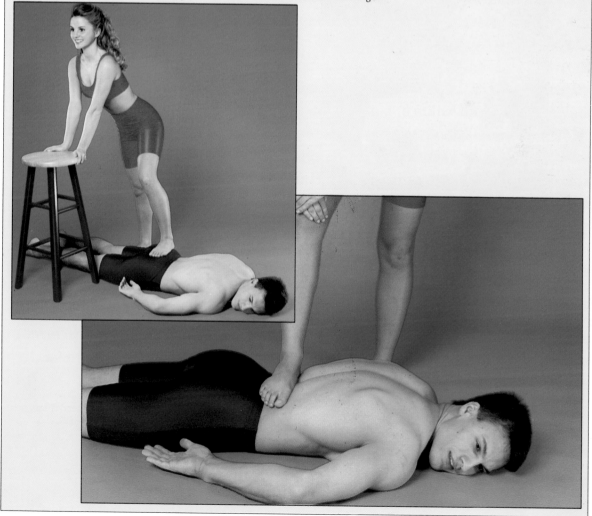

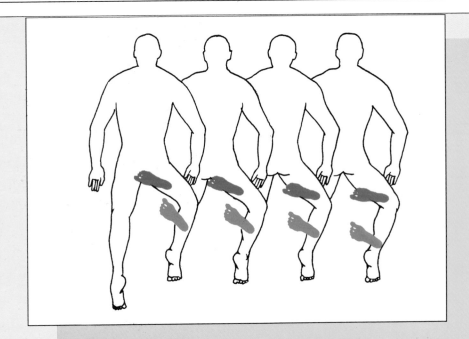

Bend the Receiver's knee slightly and repeat on the other leg and thigh.

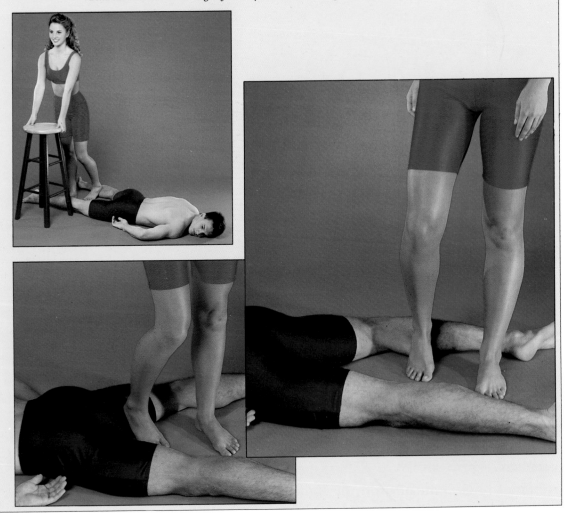

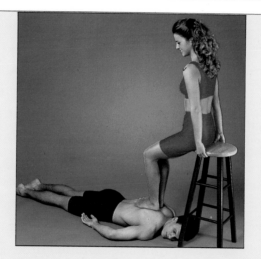

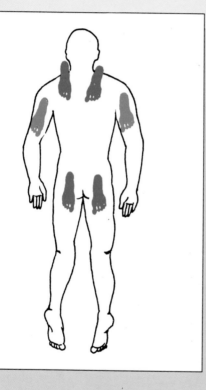

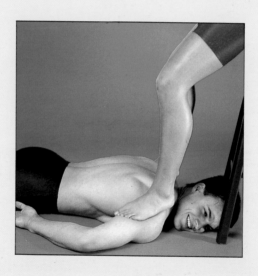

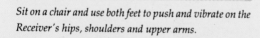

Sit on a chair and use both feet to push and vibrate on the Receiver's hips, shoulders and upper arms.

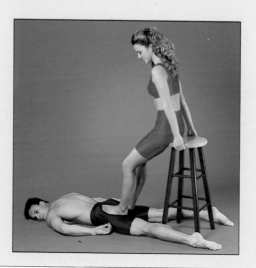

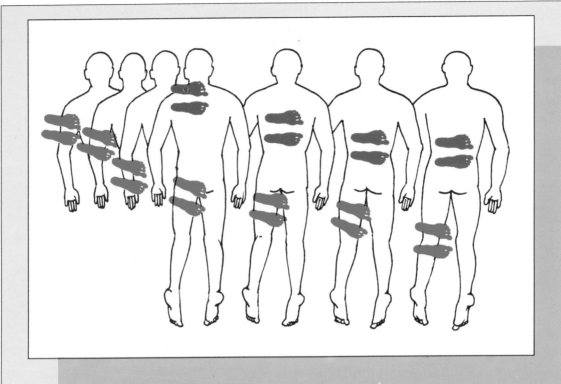

Sit on a chair and use both feet to push and vibrate on the Receiver's hips, shoulders, back, arms, legs and thighs. Repeat the process on the opposite side.

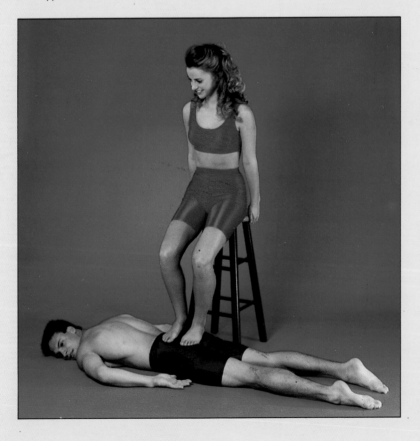

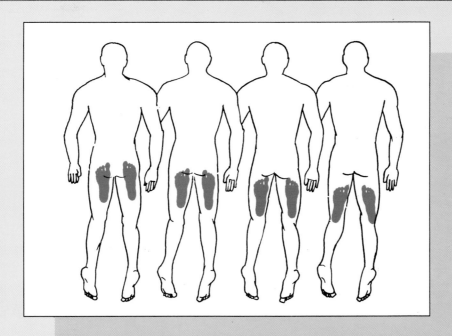

Using a chair to support your weight and to control weight and balance, gently step onto the Receiver's hips. Stand and march in place for approximately one minute before stepping onto the floor. Repeat the process on the hamstrings.

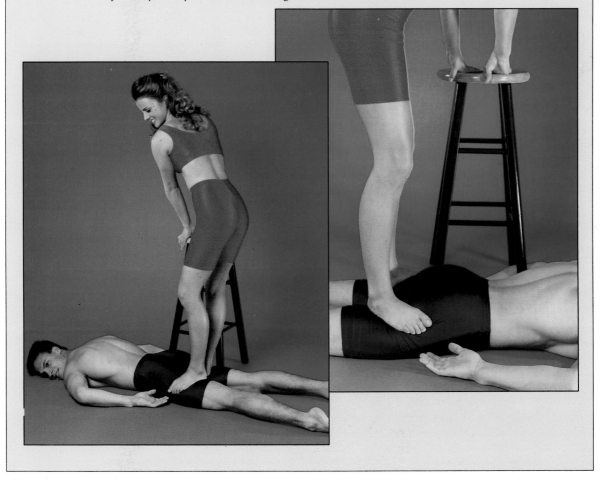

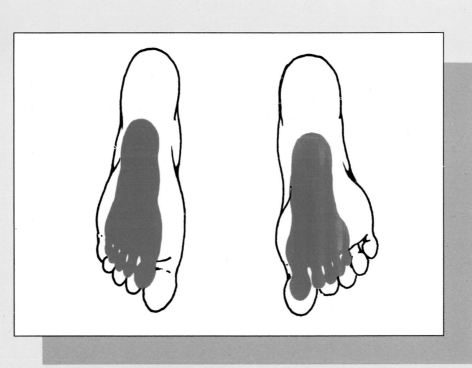

Stand and march gently on both Receiver's feet.

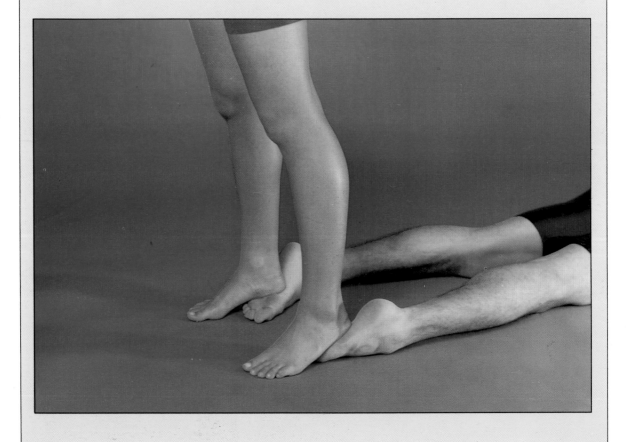

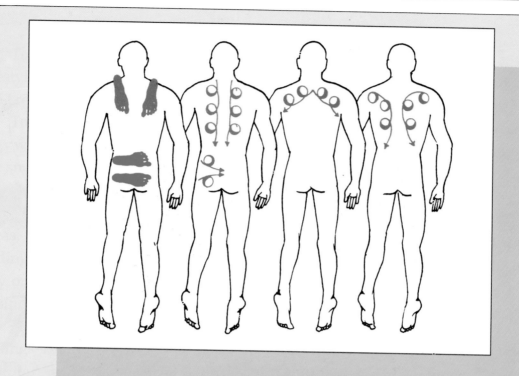

Sit on a chair and rhythmically alternate heels of both feet to massage and apply moderate pressure with an outward circular motion.

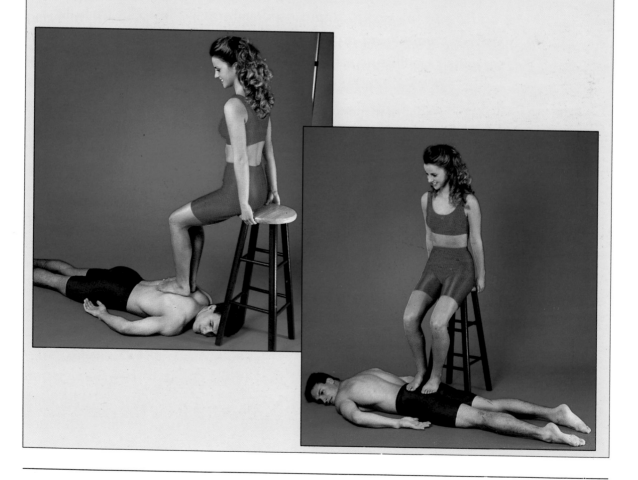

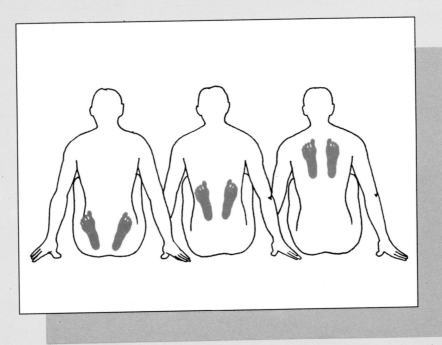

Sit behind the Receiver. Use both feet to apply moderate pressure with outward circular motion.

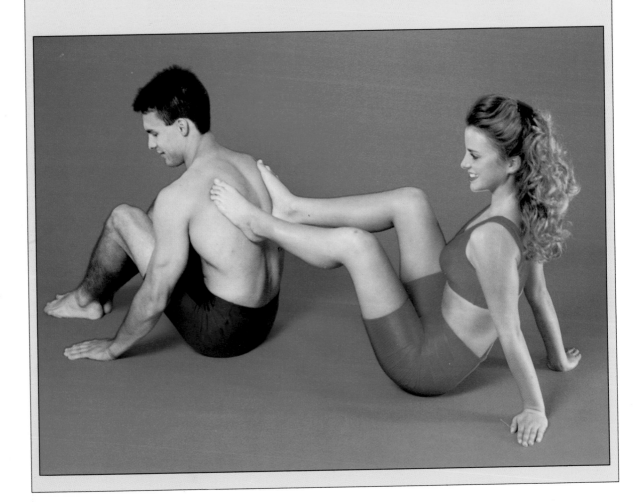

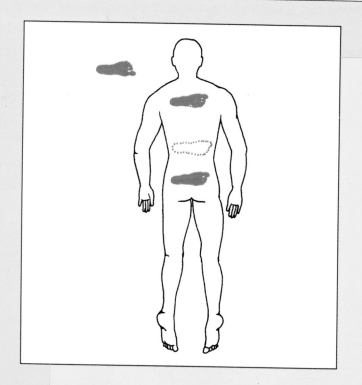

Apply oil to Receiver's back. Using a chair to support your weight and control balance, gently place the right foot onto the Receiver's upper back. Apply between 70 and 100 pounds of pressure and gently slide down the back. Repeat as many times as desired.

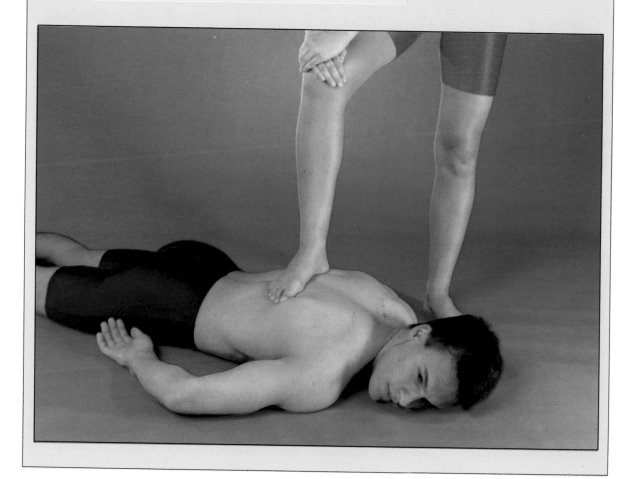

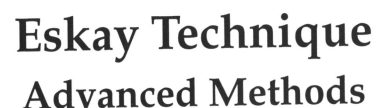

Chapter 4

Eskay Technique
Advanced Methods
Massage Tips

$\mathcal{B}$efore beginning therapeutic massage to the problem areas, keep in mind that although muscles are tough and hard to injure, pressure applied too deep or too quickly can be extremely painful and can bruise muscle fibers, thus aggravating an injury. When muscles tense during massage, lighten pressure and depth and continue the manipulation with slower pressure graduations, allowing muscles time to warm and relax. Keep in mind that muscular strength and pain tolerance differ with each individual. With practice and experience this task will grow easier--it's a judgment call.

If an area has been recently injured, do not massage directly on that area. Apply ice treatments and wait until the injured area is no longer swollen. Ice dulls peripheral pain and relieves spasm by decreasing muscle activity and lowering activity in peripheral, uninjured cells. This puts cells in partial hibernation and extension of injury is prevented. Ice should be placed in a leak-proof bag and applied to the injury for about 20 minutes, then removed for 10 minutes to prevent reflex vasocilation. This sequence of application and removal can be repeated several times during the first 24 to 48 hours. After inflammation has subsided, treat the area with light massage.

Before applying aggressive massage techniques to areas adjoining trigger points, muscles need to be warmed-up and stretched extensively. Be sure to massage the underlying tissue and not just the surface skin. Increase pressure gradually--to the verge of discomfort--with medium force for approximately 20 seconds. The force should be applied until discomfort is alleviated, then gradually increase pressure. Trigger points are sensitive to manipulation. Initially, as manipulation deepens, sensitivity will increase. As tenderness of trigger points abates, pressure can be applied for longer periods of time. And finally, don't discontinue massage when the aches and pain are gone. Frequent or daily massage can be therapeutic and preventative.

Unfortunately, some massage techniques have been commercialized to the extent that they are ineffective--nothing more than superficial physical manipulation. This does little more than produce short-term benefits and automated surface movements. Traditional massage techniques, however, have the responsibility to provide more than "improved technique" and the goal of the Eskay Technique is to produce the following:

- Relaxation, sleep and rest are enhanced through the release of specific brain chemicals called beta-endorphins or enkephalins, which are the body's naturally recurring painkillers and tranquilizers.

- Physiological and psychological stress is reduced efficiently and immediately through body-works and the release of brain chemicals and accompanying relaxation.

- Concentration is improved due to the body's enhanced relaxation, sleep, rest and recuperative abilities.

- Flexibility and mobility are improved due to the reduction of muscle hypertonicity (prolonged tension of muscle and tendons).

- Hyperemia (extra supply of blood and oxygen) production is increased due to actual physical manipulations. It aids the metabolism/combustion process that allows muscles to perform at peak physiological efficiency.

- Lymphatic performance is improved, reducing the retention of toxins and metabolites in the musculatory system, such as lactic, carbonic and uric acids.

- Edema (inflammatory agent) is reduced so the muscles can combat adhesions, soreness, swelling, cramping and spasm while encouraging sluggish circulatory systems to perform at a quicker pace.

- Overall balance and muscle control are improved, enabling musculatory systems to operate at increased levels of efficiency and encouraging the promotion of free-flowing energy.

- Recovery time is shortened because muscles are properly conditioned and the body is better prepared to respond to natural, internal healing chemicals.

Developing Massage Tools

The proper use of body "tools," the hands, can make the difference between a powerful therapeutic massage and a superficial massage. The greatest results are realized only after precise skills are mastered. The naturally simplistic, yet detailed, methods shown in this book employ innate energy to its highest advantage. In this case the simple mode is the most effective mode. Therefore, it is imperative that all students of massage concentrate on, strengthening and eventually perfecting their natural healing tools and technique.

Exercise 1

To develop thumb and finger strength, practice massaging a racquetball or squash ball every day for one hour. Racketballs or squashballs are best because of their size, shape and texture. The following exercise will accustom you to directing strength to

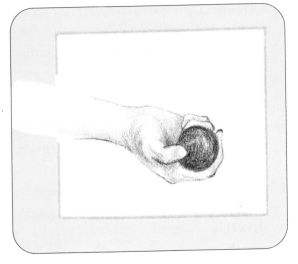

the tips of your fingers. After a few days, you will begin to notice a dramatic increase in strength and greater control of the fingers, thumb and hands. While massaging the ball with your thumbs, fingers and hands, concentrate on keeping your arms and shoulders relaxed. When you apply fingertip pressure to the ball, your body will naturally tense. To avoid this tension, mentally force your arms and shoulder to relax while maintaining finger pressure.

Begin massaging the ball with your right hand, switch to the left hand and then use both hands simultaneously. Work every muscle by changing hand and finger positions.

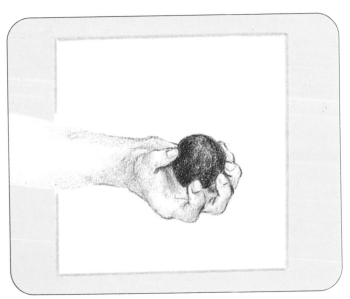

Exercise 2

This exercise was developed to perfect strength control and energy diversion. It may seem unnatural at first, but with practice you will soon be able to divert precise strength to the tips of your fingers and you will develop "super fingers."

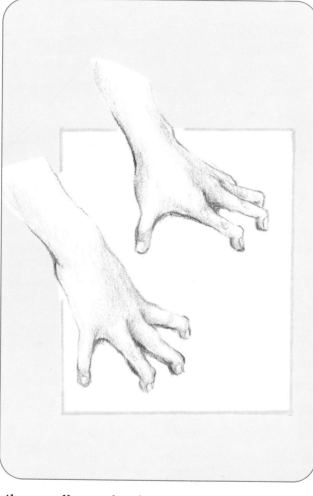

Near the tips of your fingers are seldom-used knuckles, comprising of the fingertips and fingernails, usually used only by "double-jointed" people. This knuckle, which looks quite unnatural when flexed,

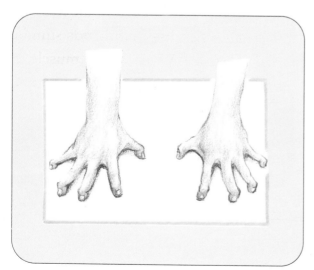

will help you achieve precise finger control.

Begin the exercise by sitting on a surface that will provide resistance for your fingers, such as a carpeted floor or rug. Using both hands simultaneously, open your fingers wide and place the tips of your fingers on the floor in front of you. Pretend the floor is a piano keyboard. Push against your fingertip knuckle but keep your fingers straight. Only the tips of your fingers are bent. Push hard and hold your position. Use your body weight to increase pressure and push against your fingertip knuckle for one minute. Next, pull your flexed fingers toward you and repeat the process. The pulling effect creates strength in the tips of your fingers.

TECHNIQUE
The Scorpion Technique

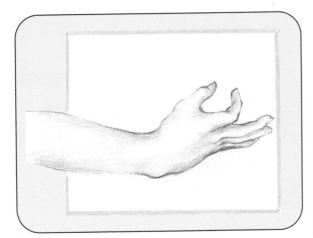

healthy, therapeutic technique. In massage, the Scorpion Technique is for small, precise kneading action used to reach ar-

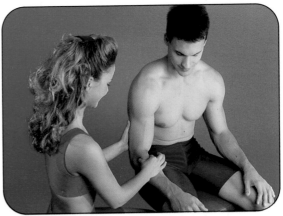

Pinch the forearm with the scorpion technique.

The Scorpion evolved from ancient Asian Martial Arts. In its original form, the "Scorpion" depended on a deadly, two-finger move used to strike vulnerable areas of an opponent's body. Ancient Masters used this knowledge and combined it with acupuncture point know-how to create a

eas between muscle and bone. It permits specific muscle areas which require deep penetration to be raised and manipulated.

The Scorpion Technique combines several gliding, circling, pinching motions into one fluid movement to create a rhythmic, hypnotic, systematic technique of pres-

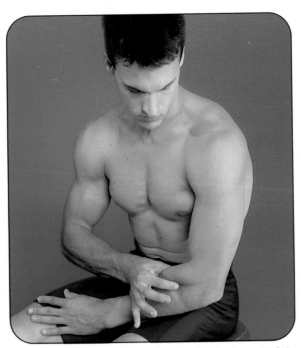

Pinch the forearm between the thumb and index finger. Use the scorpion technique to massage towards the wrist.

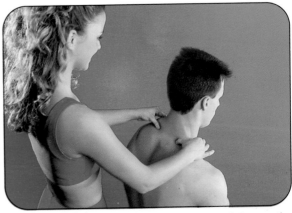

Using the scorpion technique. Nip the trapezius muscle between the finger and thumb. Massage outward toward the shoulder.

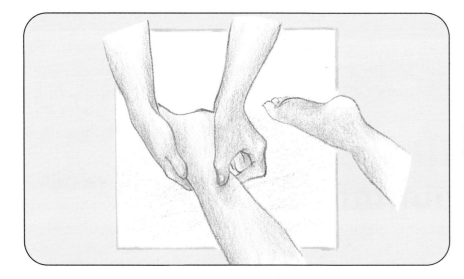

Nip the achilles tendon, massage toward the calf using the scorpion technique.

sure variations. It uses the index or middle fingers and thumbs to "pinch" or "nip" muscles in sliding, spiraling motions. Fingers should not completely lift off the body but should glide and squeeze downward, while making small elliptical circles.

Practice the Scorpion Technique on any accessible, comfortable area, such as the hands, triceps, forearms, or shoulders. On the shoulder, spiral the fingers on both hands down the muscle with small circles.

Remember to pinch and release while circling. Start a circle with pressure, release when you complete the circle, then begin the next circle while you are still gliding. Each movement should blend fluidly into the next. Do not maintain constant pressure while circling.

The Scorpion Technique separates muscle fibers that are bunched or knotted and produces soothing effects. It can be applied to any muscle of the body.

The Thumb Technique

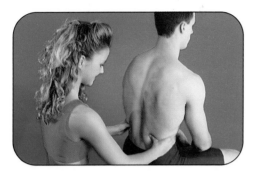

Apply thumb pressure on either side of the spine. Massage up and down the lower back.

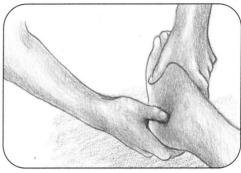

Use thumb technique to gradually increase pressure around the ankle area.

The Thumb Technique is a "knot buster" and was designed for lingering penetration. It allows precise control through shallow or deep muscle manipulation and is best for working

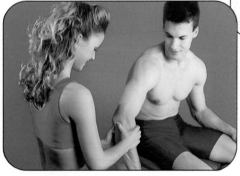

Apply deep circular pressure with thumbs on either side of the elbow.

out knots and spasms over the entire body.

The secret of this technique is to always move the thumb in small circles and to gradually increase thumb pressure to tense or knotted areas. Practice the Thumb Technique on the small muscles of the back and shoulders. These muscles can be relieved of tension and spasm by using the tips of both thumbs to apply deep, circular pressure. Work on each area for several seconds before moving on; massage knotted or tense areas until tightness subsides.

Place the thumb of each hand on either

side of the spine at the base of the neck. Using the tips of your thumbs, make small, moderately deep circles in one long spiral down the edges of the spine. Now, beginning at the top of the shoulders, repeat the Thumb Technique down the shoulder blade to work out

Use thumb technique to apply deep circular pressure around trigger points of the lower back. Be sure to avoid direct pressure to the spine.

tight areas. If knots persist, work on them with gentle, deep, circular motions. Begin with a light stroke and increase pressure until the tightness subsides. If knots still persist, repeat the technique using both thumbs side-by-side to the tense area. Continue treatment as long as necessary.

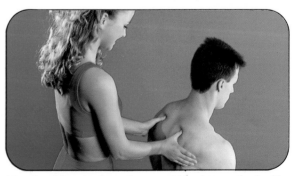

Move thumb in a circular motion up and down between the shoulder blades.

The Palm Technique

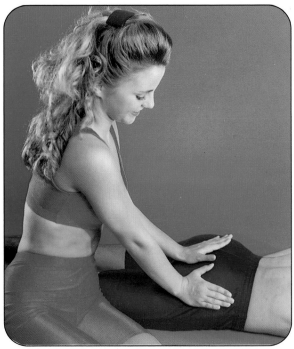

Using the palm technique, alternate pressure between the hands to massage the hips and buttock muscles.

The Palm Technique was developed for areas of great sensitivity. The sciatic nerve, the largest nerve in the body, takes root in the lower spine and runs down both legs. Sensitive areas, such as the buttocks, become painful because of tension in this nerve. The Palm Technique allows sensitive areas to be manipulated without causing further tension to the receiver.

Begin with your wrists together, then use the balls of your palms to apply moderate pressure with outward circular mo-

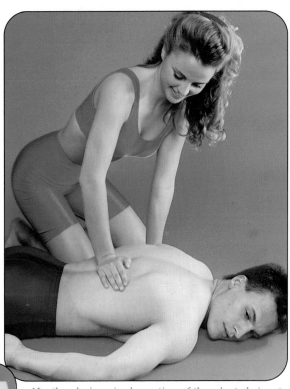

Use the relaxing, circular motions of the palm technique to relieve tense back muscles.

tions. Practice this technique on the buttocks.

Other techniques designed to relax the buttocks, although effective, often cause discomfort. Tensing or tightness from discomfort will minimize the effectiveness of manipulation.

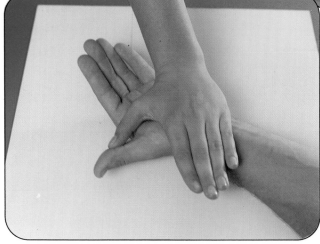

Press your palm in an outward circular motion increase depth gradually.

The Knuckle and Elbow Technique

The Knuckle and Elbow Techniques were developed for hard-to-reach or fleshy areas. They are optional techniques that allow deeper penetration than the Scorpion or Thumb techniques.

In both techniques circular and gliding motions are used to relieve muscle knots and spasms, and body weight is added to increase depth and pressure with minimal effort by Giver and maximum relief for the Receiver.

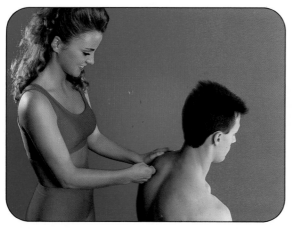

Apply knuckle pressure on trigger points around the shoulder blade.

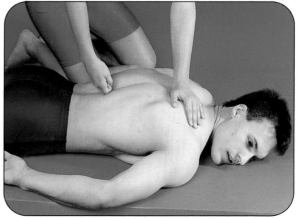

Use the knuckle technique to massage the back muscles in penetrating circular motions.

The Knuckle Technique

The Knuckle Technique is a combination of pressure-circular and pressure-gliding movements. With the fingers bent at the middle knuckles practice the Knuckle Technique on the shoulders and between the shoulders and vertebrae. Find knots in these areas and relieve them with the circular Knuckle Technique. As the knot softens, increase pressure by using body weight to gently "lean" into the muscle until the knot or spasm is released.

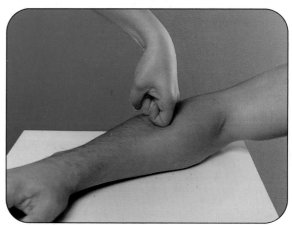

Use knuckle to apply circular pressure across the muscles of the forearm.

The Elbow Technique

The Elbow Technique has been called, "the lazy man's technique", because it is easy and requires minimum effort. Although effective, the Elbow Technique can be insensitive to depth and knotted areas. Givers should be aware of the Receiver's comfort. The Elbow Technique should be used on large muscles, such as areas around the vertebrae, shoulders, lower back and thighs. Similar to the Knuckle Technique, the Elbow Technique relies on circular and gliding motions.

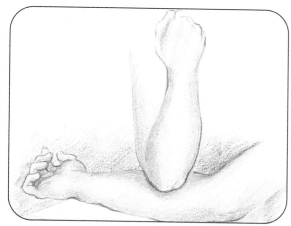

Use elbow technique to massage the muscles of the forearm.

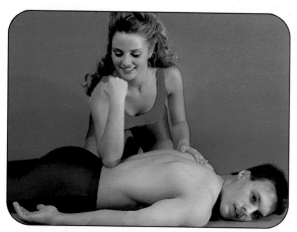

Use body weight to deeply massage the muscles of the lower back in a circular motion. Avoid the spine.

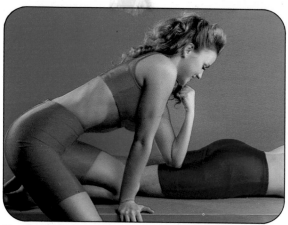

Use elbow technique on large hamstring muscles. Increase pressure gradually by applying body weight.

Practice the gliding-elbow technique on the large muscle areas or the back. Glide down on either side of the vertebrae from the shoulder to the waist.

Use the bent elbow to "point" to the aggravated muscle or muscle group in pain or spasm. Apply circular, gliding movements, using body weight to increase pressure and to penetrate deeper into the muscle. Practice the gliding Elbow Technique on the large muscle areas of the back. Glide down on either side of the vertebrae from the shoulder to the waist.

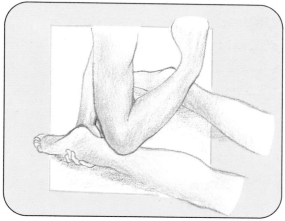

Use elbow to massage the archilles tendon.

The Kneading Technique

The Kneading Technique is universally known and practiced—and it works wonders. At one time or another, you have probably kneaded sore areas of your own body. Similar to kneading dough, this technique involves grasping flesh alternately between thumb and forefingers in a rhythmic pattern.

Practice this technique on the Receiver's arms. With both hands, gently but firmly grasp the Receiver's arm between thumbs and forefingers. Without lifting your hands, squeeze and release the flesh in one hand and then squeeze and release the flesh in the other hand. Rhythmically alternate hands. As one hand releases flesh, the other hand grabs a handful of flesh nearby.

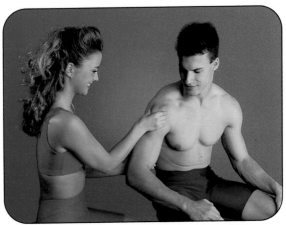

Knead the Receiver's shoulder before applying deeper pressure on trigger points.

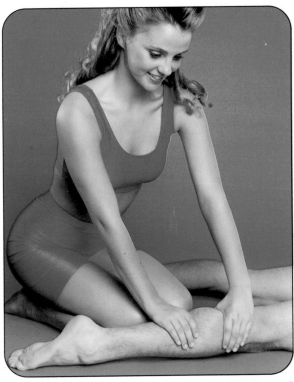

With both hands knead the calf muscles. Pressure should be alternated between the hands.

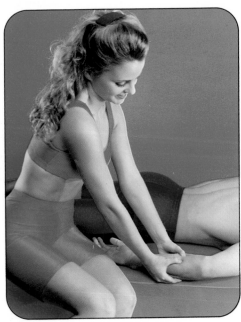

Use both hands to knead the forearm.

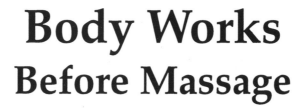

Chapter 5

Body Works
Before Massage

The Giver

- Be healthy. Never massage when you are ill or weak.
- Trim nails and cuticles so they are short and smooth. Long fingernails will restrict you from using many techniques.
- Wear loose-fitting clothing that enables you to move freely and comfortably.

The Receiver

- Don't allow yourself to be massaged if you have a high fever or if your skin is irritated or infected.
- Wear loose fitting clothing, minimal clothing, or no clothing at all. Be comfortable.
- Surrender yourself to the Giver's hands and allow your body to totally relax.
- Communicate your comfort or discomfort to the Giver.

Remember: Unlike other massage disciplines, it is not necessary to perform all manipulations illustrated here. Any of these massage techniques or positions can be used singly to ease tightness or discomfort in a specific muscle area. All are shown for reference, but each can be used separately and/or in any sequence.

Trigger Point Massage

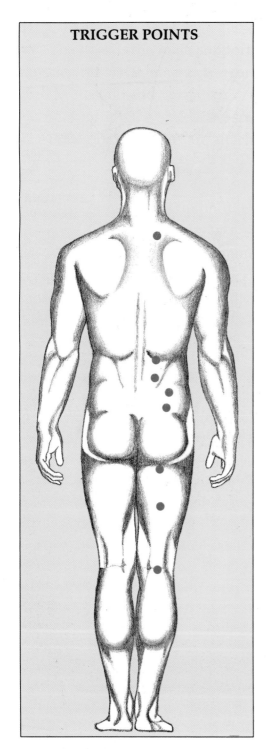

TRIGGER POINTS

When beginning massage, the Giver should start with light strokes, such as with palm or kneading techniques. The Giver should allow the Receiver's body to grow accustomed to his/her touch. The Giver should be aware of the Receiver's comfort and ask for feedback. As the Receiver relaxes, the Giver may begin to increase depth and pressure gradually, without severe discomfort or muscle tension. As the Receiver warms up, the Giver may begin working on knots or trigger points, tensed or areas in spasm by using the thumb, knuckle, elbow, or scorpion techniques to make small, moderately deep circles.

The most important element of trigger point massage is to move the thumb, knuckle and elbow in small circles and gradually increase pressure. As the Receiver grows more comfortable, the Giver may apply constant pressure (up to 30 lbs. for 30 seconds) to the trigger point area. This pressure, applied with moderate force, should inactivate the muscle area. The Giver may use the thumb, elbow and knuckle techniques directly on the trigger point.

If the trigger points are tender, the Giver should apply pressure for only a second or two. As the point or area becomes less tender, the receiver will be able to withstand more pressure for longer periods of time. Tenderness usually indicates that treatment is needed. Diminished tenderness indicates successful treatment. If knots persist, the Giver should continue applying deep, gentle circular pressure to the areas until they are loosened and pain subsides.

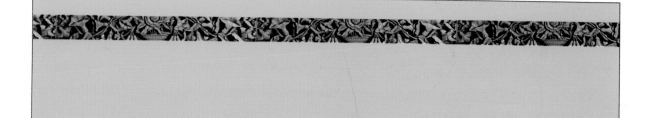

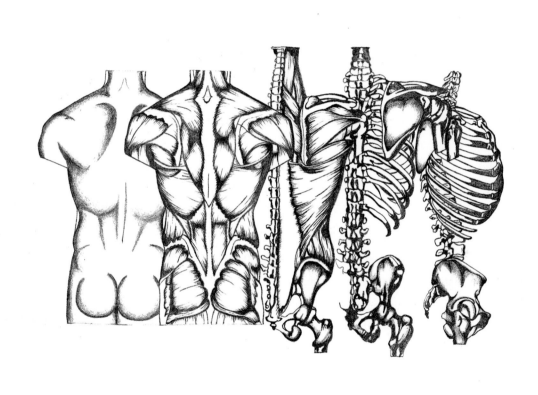

THE BACK

The Back

The back is the main supportive framework for the body. Made up of vertebrae, muscles, nerves, ligaments and cartilages, the back provides upper body support, spinal cord protection and flexibility.

Supporting the back is the spinal column, made up of 24 vertically stacked bones. The bones, or vertebrae, are attached to each other by spongy discs which act as shock absorbers.

Behind the vertebrae lies a protected canal of arched bone, which protects the spinal cord. The spinal cord is a conduit for sending messages from the brain to the limbs and back to the brain.

The spinal column rests in three natural curves: cervical, thoracic and lumbar. The cervical spine supports the neck and allows mobility; the thoracic spine has little mobility but supports the middle back and protects the lungs; and the lumbar spine supports the lower back and contains the strongest and largest vertebrae. When all three curves are in normal position, the body is balanced and body weight is evenly distributed.

Many common back problems stem from years of abuse. Poor posture, obesity, weak muscles, improper lifting, poor sleeping surfaces or positions, sitting and standing take the body out of its natural alignment. Many back problems can be corrected effortlessly, but others take special care and supervision.

Posture determines the proper alignment of vertebrae. When slumped or slouched, the back is forced into unnatural positions. These awkward positions promote vertebrae and ligament irregularities which cause back pain. When good posture is practiced, body weight is evenly distributed. Even, balanced weight distribution relieves pressure constantly put on muscles.

Try to keep the back in a position that maintains the natural curvature of the spine. Use abdominal and buttock muscles to maintain comfort, and change positions often. Excess body weight pulls the spine out of balance. Weak, flabby stomach and back muscles greatly increase the incidence of permanent imbalance or injury, however, see a health professional for assistance before initiating weight loss.

Similar to the effects of extra body weight, weak back, hip, buttock, and leg muscles shift the spine and the three natural curves. Neglected muscles provide poor dynamic support to the spine and invite injury. By strengthening these muscle groups, the spine will be adequately supported and proper body alignment will be maintained.

Sitting incorrectly for long periods can place stress on the spine. Choose a chair that supports the back or use a pillow or a rolled towel for added comfort and to reduce stress to the spine.

When sitting or standing, keep both feet flat on the floor and stretch periodically. Occasionally, prop one foot on a box or low stool. When standing, try to keep the body in a natural, balanced position.

Common back complaint, such as lower back pain, muscle spasm, sprains, and strains are frequently attributed to the problems discussed above. By strengthening back, leg and buttock muscles, concentrating on good posture, maintaining ideal weight and learning the proper ways to lift, sit and stand, many common back ailments can be eliminated.

Lower Back Pain
General Massage Areas

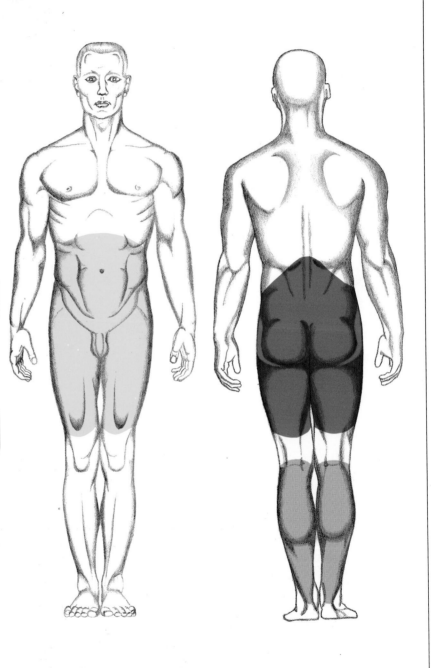

**Maximum
Pressure**

**35 LBS
25 LBS**

**Moderate
Pressure**

**25 LBS
15 LBS**

**Minimum
Pressure**

**15 LBS
5 LBS**

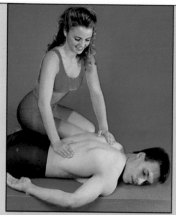

Use palm technique to apply gradually increasing pressure. This allows the muscles to relax.

The thumb can be used to apply gradually increasing pressure to trigger point areas.

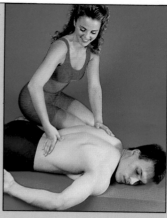

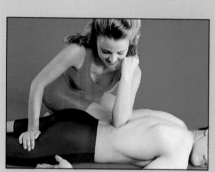

Use bodyweight to control depth of elbow pressure. Be aware of Receiver's comfort level.

TRIGGER POINTS

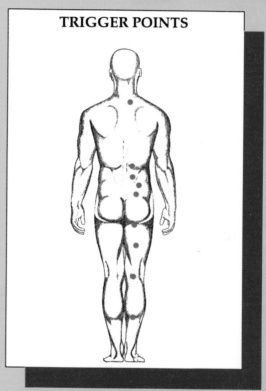

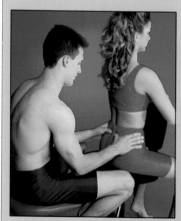

Receiver sit on a chair. Giver apply thumb technique to Receiver's low to mid-back.

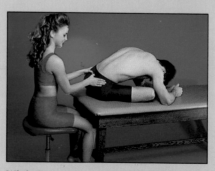

While Receiver is in a stretch position, use thumb technique to work on trigger points around lower back.

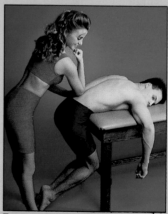

For maximum release to spasms around lower back, use elbow technique on the stretched lower back

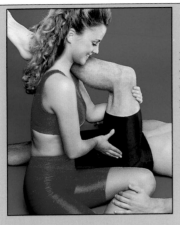

Rest the Receiver's leg on your shoulder. Use thumb technique to massage the hamstring trigger points.

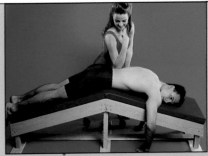

For added pressure, use elbow technique to work on trigger points around the lower back.

TRIGGER POINTS

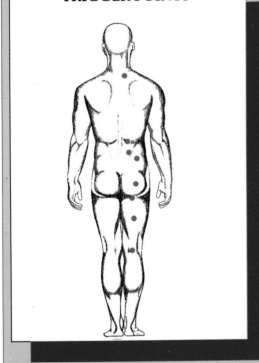

With Receiver bent at waist, use elbow technique on stretched lower back muscles and trigger points.

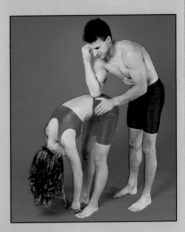

Place thumbs on the muscles on either side of the spine. Massage up and down the lower back muscles.

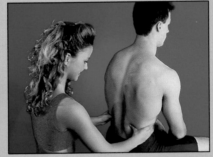

While Receiver is stretching the calf and hamstring, manipulate trigger points around the back of the knee.

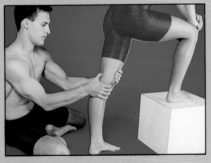

For convenience, in a stance position use thumb technique on Receiver's hamstring.

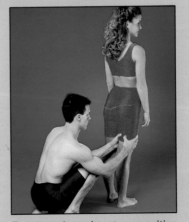

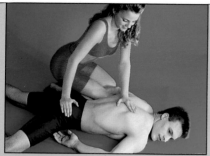

Position the Receiver with one leg bent and apply pressure to the hip area using the palm technique.

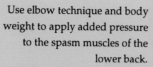

Use elbow technique and body weight to apply added pressure to the spasm muscles of the lower back.

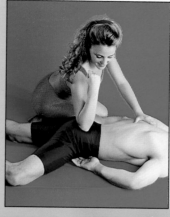

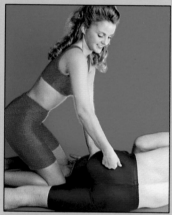

Use thumb technique on trigger points around Receiver's sacro-iliac joint.

TRIGGER POINTS

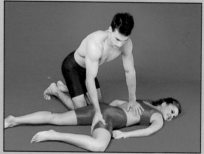

Use thumb technique to apply deep circular pressure on trigger points on ilio-tibial band.

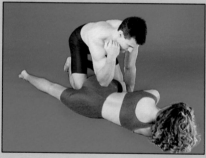

Receiver on side and leg bent. Use elbow to work on spasms around piriformis muscles and sacro-iliac joint.

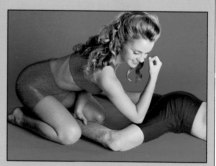

Use elbow technique on Receiver's ilio-tibial band (I.T. Band) trigger points.

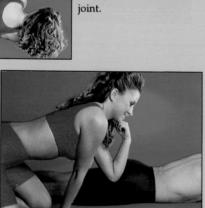

Use elbow technique to work around the trigger point areas of the upper leg (Hamstring) and buttocks.

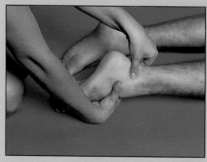

Nip Receiver's achilles tendon using the scorpion technique. Massage up towards the calf.

BACK PROBLEM
S T R E T C H I N G

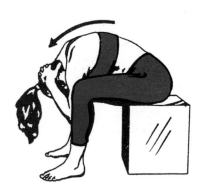

BACK CURL
Sitting on bench as shown, curl back forward with neck relaxed. Hold five seconds, then slowly return to seated position. Repeat three times.

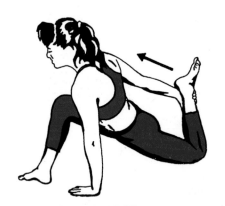

THE ATHLETIC QUAD STRETCH
Kneel on one knee, front leg at 90 degree angle as shown. With right hand grasp left foot, slowly lower front hip toward floor while gently pulling ankle toward buttocks. Hold 20 seconds. Repeat three times on each side.

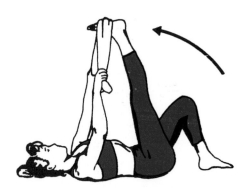

HAMSTRING STRETCH
Lying on floor, one knee bent as shown, loop towel around other foot. Tighten stomach muscles and raise leg up until slight tightness is felt. Keep knee joint locked and pull towards the head. Repeat three times with each leg.

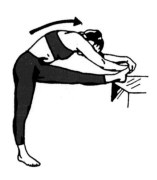

ATHLETIC HAMSTRING STRETCH
Stand erect with heel on counter or barre about hip height. Slowly roll upper body forward; place hands on foot, calf, or thigh. Hold stretch 20 seconds. Repeat three times with each leg.

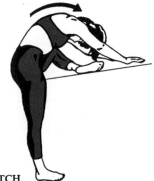

PIRIFORMIS STRETCH
Position body with one leg bent on counter or barre as shown. Curl upper body over bent leg and reach arms forward. Hold, then repeat three times with each leg.

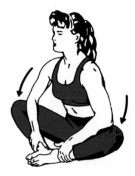

SITTING ADDUCTOR STRETCH
Sitting with soles of feet together, grasp ankles and press legs toward floor with elbows as shown. Hold stretch 20 seconds and release. If back is uncomfortable or tight, move feet away from body. Repeat three times.

BACK PROBLEM
S T R E T C H I N G

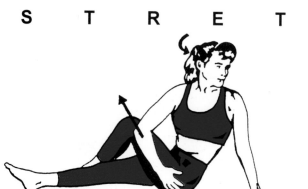

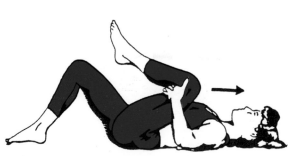

SPINAL TWIST

Sitting on floor with one leg crossed as shown, rotate upper body in direction of bent leg. Push against crossed leg until stretch is felt. Use free arm and elbow to press against leg to increase stretch. Hold stretch for 10 seconds. Repeat three times on each side.

KNEE TO CHEST

Lie on back with both legs bent as shown. Grasp leg behind knee with both hands and pull toward chest. Press lower back against floor. Hold, then repeat three times on each leg.

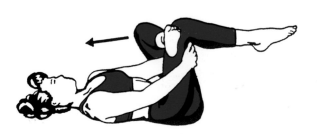

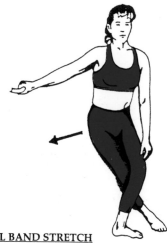

HIP ROTATORS

Lie on back with foot resting on knee. Grasp thigh behind knee with both hands and pull toward chest as shown. Hold stretch 20 seconds. Do not bounce. Repeat three times on each side.

ILIOTIBIAL BAND STRETCH

Standing with one hand holding the counter or barre for support and stability as shown, position one leg behind the other and push hips toward supporting hand. Feel the stretch along the outside of the thigh. Hold for 20 seconds, then repeat three times on each side. Do not bounce.

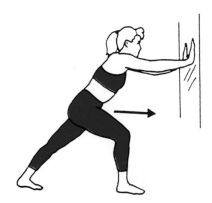

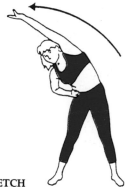

CALF STRETCH

Standing at wall with one foot back 3-4 feet from wall, opposite knee bent, lean against wall with hands. Lower hips until stretch is felt. Hold for 20 seconds, then repeat three times on each leg. Keep back leg straight, heels flat.

TRUNK STRETCH

Reach up and out with your arm. Feel the stretch in your side and arm. Keep your knee slightly bent. Hold for 20 seconds. Repeat three times on each side.

BACK PROBLEM
S   T   R   E   T   C   H   I   N   G

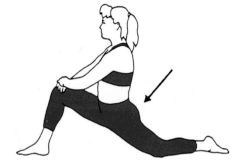

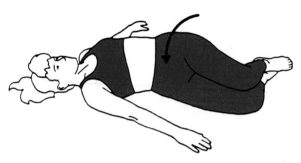

HIP STRETCH

Kneel on floor with front knee bent at 90 degree angle and back leg extended. Tighten stomach muscles and shift weight forward on front foot. Hold stretch 20 seconds, then repeat three times on each side.

Trunk Roll

Lying on back with knees bent, feet flat, rotate hips and drop knees to one side. Keep shoulders and hand flat on the floor. Hold for 10 seconds. Return to starting position and repeat three times on each side.

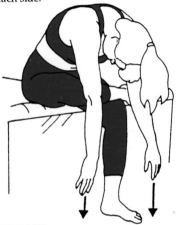

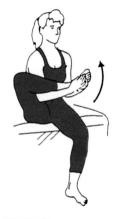

CHAIR STRETCH

Sit on edge of chair or bench, one knee bent with ankle resting on opposite leg as shown. Roll back forward and stretch arms toward the floor. Hold for 20 seconds, then return to starting position. Repeat three times on each side.

SITTING YOGA STRETCH

Sit erect on chair or bench, one leg crossed the other. Cradle bent leg in arms and pull upward chest, keeping back straight. Hold stretch for 10 seconds, then repeat three times on each side.

BACK PROBLEM
S T R E N G T H E N I N G

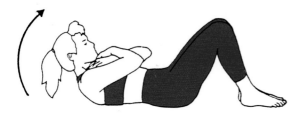

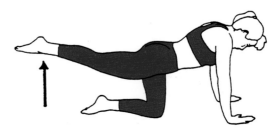

PARTIAL SIT-UP

Lying on back with knees bent, feet flat, arms crossed as shown, tuck chin toward chest and lift head and shoulders off floor. Using your stomach muscles "crunch" then return to floor. Do not hold breath. Repeat 10 times.

QUADRIPED

Beginning on hands and knees, back straight, extend one leg back. Elevate ankle slightly to increase stretch, then return to starting position. Progressively increase your hold. Repeat 10 times on each side.

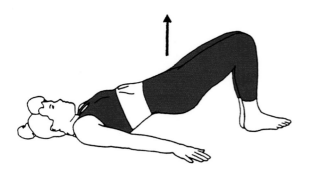

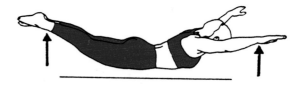

BRIDGING

Lying on back with knees bent, feet flat, tighten buttocks muscles and lift hips, back and buttocks off the floor. Hold 10 seconds. Repeat 10 times.

ATHLETIC BACK EXTENSION

Lying face down on floor, arms and legs extended, arch back to simultaneously lift upper body and legs upward. Hold five seconds then release. Repeat 10 times.

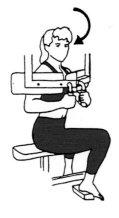

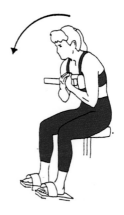

ROTARY TORSO

Adjust weight, angle of torsion, and seat height. Press chest firmly against chest pad, grasp handles, and turn to one side. Exhale as you slowly turn to the other side. Control the machine's return; do not let the weights slam together on return. Do three of 10 repetitions. Progressively increase your weights.

ABDOMINAL

Adjust weight, seat and leg height, and position arms as shown. Exhale as you lean forward, leading with the chest. Tighten stomach muscles to keep movements slow. Do not let weights slam together on return. Do three sets of 10 repetitions. Progressively increase your weights.

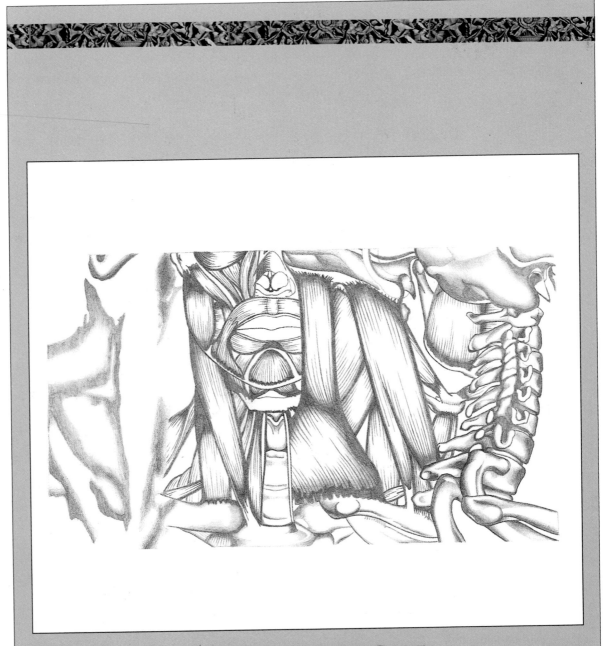

THE NECK

The Neck

The neck, or cervical spine, consists of seven vertebrae, connected by shock-absorbing discs. The cervical spine allows head and neck movements, and helps support and balance the head. Strong neck and shoulder muscles support the spine and increase flexibility.

The spinal cord, nerves and blood vessels course through the neck. Branches of nerves from the spinal cord send messages to the head, shoulders, chest and arms allowing movement and sensation.

Common neck problems include strains, sprains, tears, arthritis, and herniated discs. Common culprits are stress, poor posture, inadequate sleeping positions or surface, and normal wear and tear.

Sprains, strains and tears occur when muscles and ligaments are stretched beyond their normal range of motion. Commonly known as "whiplash", sprains and strains usually occur when a snapping motion causes the body to try to move one way and the head the other. Although symptoms vary, most whiplash victims complain of neck pain and stiffness.

Occasionally tennis players suffer from "wryneck" which is characterized by the ability to move the head only in one direction. Sometimes an overhead smash pulls a muscle or causes muscle spasm.

Another localized muscle spasm caused by pulling or damaging fibers in the trapezius muscle is known as "trapezius triggers". The spasm causes a reflex in which the nerve fibers fire, the muscle contracts, and a sensation of pain is felt. The impulse causes other nerve fibers to fire, more muscle contraction, etc. Ice treatments to the neck, and massage to stretch the muscle gives relief.

Poor posture leads to neck problems by pulling the weight of the head off centered. When the head and neck are off centered, the spine is forced out of its natural curves. Neck muscles contract, are fatigued and cause pain. Awkward sleeping positions, large pillows or flat, soft surface also strain the neck, stress the spine, and contribute to neck pain.

As we age, so does the cervical spine. Discs which separate vertebrae wear and lose much of their cushioning ability. Worn discs rupture (or herniate) and press on nerves.

Except for normal wear and tear, most neck problems can be prevented, improved or eliminated with a common-sense approach to neck health. Maintain the body's three natural spinal curves by strengthening neck, back and abdominal muscle to alleviate neck pain and tension. In addition, athletes should improve neck strength with basic resistance exercises. A program of stretching and strengthening, stress management, a firm mattress, a low pillow, and good posture will keep the neck and spine strong and flexible.

Neck Pain And Whiplash
General Massage Areas

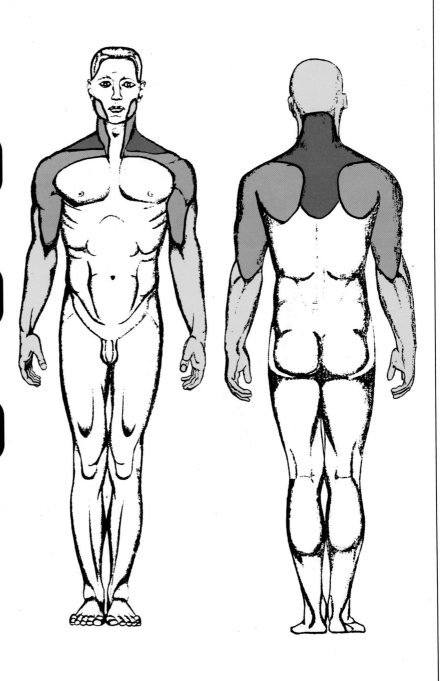

Maximum Pressure

35 LBS
25 LBS

Moderate Pressure

25 LBS
15 LBS

Minimum Pressure

15 LBS
5 LBS

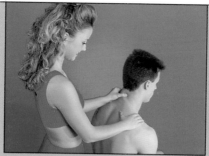

Head forward, use the thumb technique to work on the stretch neck muscles.

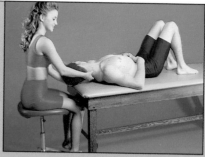

While one hand is holding the Receiver's head and neck, stretch it to the side. Use thumb technique on the trigger points of the neck.

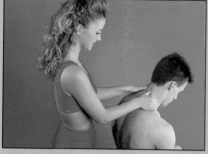

Head forward, apply thumb technique of both hands along the muscles of the neck.

TRIGGER POINTS

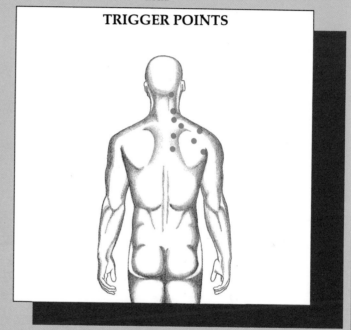

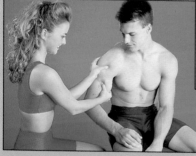

Using the scorpion technique nip the trapezius muscles between the finger and thumb. Massage outward toward the shoulder.

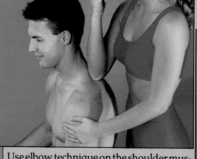

Use elbow technique on the shoulder muscles and trigger points

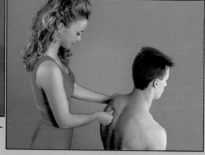

Use thumb technique to work on trigger points along the shoulder blade.

Knead from the shoulder to the elbow using both hands.

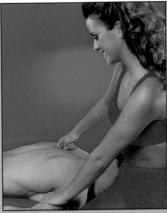

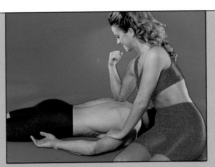

Use elbow to make small circular motions on Receiver's back. Avoid the spine.

Use knuckle to work on trigger points of Receiver's back.

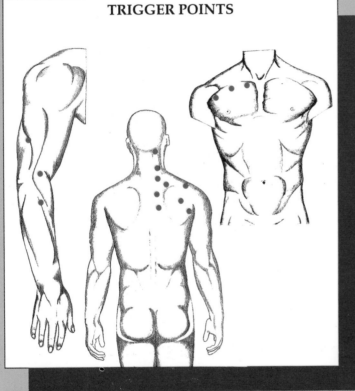

TRIGGER POINTS

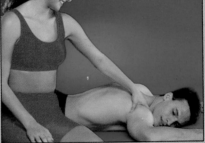

Apply thumb technique to Receiver's muscles around the arm pit.

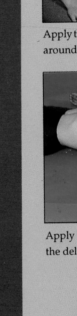

Apply thumb technique on trigger points on the deltoid and pectoral muscles.

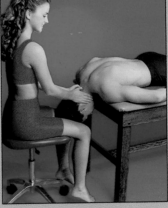

Use the fingers of both hands, lift the head and massage the base of the neck.

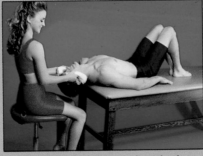

Use a towel to gently stretch and release Receiver's neck -Hold for 10 seconds.

Have Receiver carefully hang head forward so that neck is stretched. Use thumb technique on trigger points of the neck.

NECK

S T R E T C H I N G

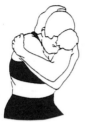

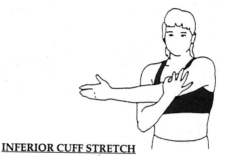

RHOMBOID STRETCH

Wrap arms around chest and grab shoulder blades as shown. With mouth close, bring chin to chest and try to pull shoulder blades forward until slight stretch is felt. Hold 10 to 20 seconds. Repeat 3 times.

INFERIOR CUFF STRETCH

Standing as shown, grasp arm just above elbow and gently pull elbow toward body. Hold 10 to 20 seconds. Repeat 3 times with each arm.

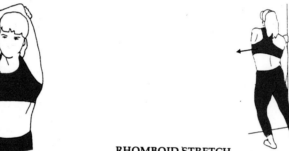

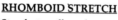

POSTERIOR CUFF STRETCH

Standing as shown, raise arm over head and grasp arm near elbow. Pull arm toward body until gentle stretch is felt and hold 20 seconds. Repeat 3 times with each arm.

RHOMBOID STRETCH

Stand at wall or doorway as shown, arm across chest, hand grasping corner, knees slightly bent. Shift weight and lean to side, until gentle stretch is felt in shoulder. Hold 20 seconds. Repeat 3 times with each arm.

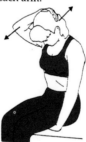

PECTORALIS STRETCH

Stand in corner with hands at shoulder level as shown. Lean forward until stretch is felt across chest. Hold 20 seconds. Repeat 3 times.

NECK FLEXION

Sitting on bench or chair as shown, reach overhead with one hand gently pull head forward and down. Hold ten seconds then return to starting position. Repeat 5 times.

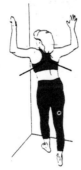

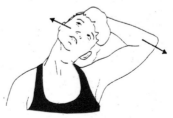

THORACIC STRETCH

Stand at bar as shown, hands shoulder-width apart, hips directly above feet. With knees slightly bent, let body drop down until slight stretch is felt in upper body and back. Bend knees a bit more or position hands at different heights to change stretch. Hold comfortable stretch 30 seconds. Repeat 3 times.

SCALENE STRETCH

Sitting upright with head tilted slightly backward and to one side, reach overhead and gently pull head downward. Hold 10 to 20 seconds. Repeat 5 times to each side.

NECK
S T R E N G T H E N I N G

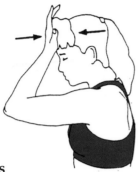

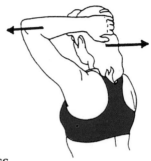

PALM PRESS
Sitting erect, head straight, press palm against forehead while resisting with neck muscles. Hold 5 second then slowly release pressure. Repeat 5 times.

PALM PRESS
Place palms of hands on back of head as shown. Press head backwards into hands while resisting with neck muscles. Hold 5 seconds then slowly release pressure. Repeat 5 times.

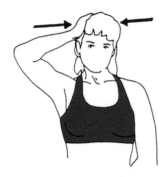

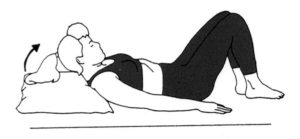

PALM PRESS
Place hand on side of head as shown. Press hand against head while resisting with neck muscles. Hold 5 seconds then slowly release pressure. Do not push against jawbone. Repeat 5 times to each side.

HEAD LIFTS
Lie on back as shown, head and neck propped on pillow, feet and hands flat. Look at ceiling, tighten neck and chest muscles, and raise and lower head off pillow. Repeat 5 times.

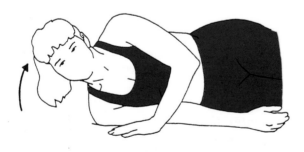

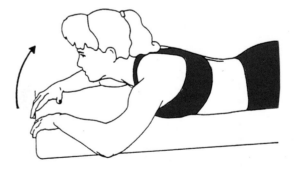

HEAD LIFTS
Lying on side as shown, one hand to front for stability, tighten neck and chest muscles to lift lower head. Repeat 5 times on each side.

HEAD LIFTS
Lie on stomach as shown hands forward or grasping edge of mat or table. Tighten neck and chest muscles and lift head toward ceiling. Repeat 5 times.

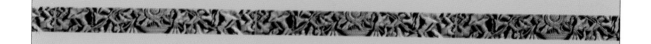

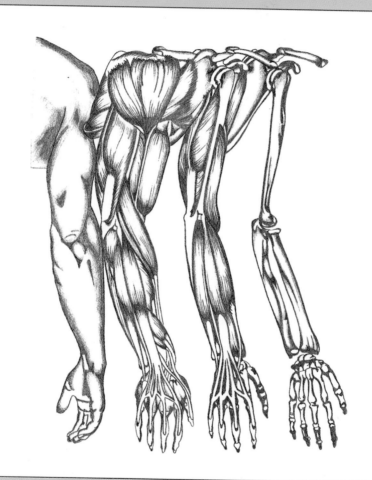

THE SHOULDER

The Shoulder

The shoulder is the most mobile joint in the body, able to rotate 360 degrees. It is the only joint not held together by ligaments--its ligaments merely keep it from moving too far in any direction. This complex structure is made up of three bones, attached by ligaments, tendons and muscle.

The first bone, the collarbone (clavicle) is a round attachment which connects the shoulder to the ribcage; the shoulder blade (scapula) connects with the collarbone and projects the upper part of the shoulder, called the acromion; the upper arm bone (humerus) joins the shoulder blade and rests in a socket of the shoulder blade known as the glennoid fossa.

The glennoid fossa socket forms part of the shoulder joint. The humerus (arm bone) fits into the fossa and is held there by a collection of muscles called the rotator cuff. The rotator cuff originates on the shoulder blade and inserts on the humerus. The bicep's tendons also connect the shoulder joint and upper arm.

Due to the lack of ligaments and a shallow socket, weakness in the rotator cuff muscles can cause the head of the shoulder to slip or to slide out of the socket in full or partial dislocation. Exercises to strengthen the rotator cuff muscles will prevent shoulder "pops" and dislocations.

Between the rotator cuff and acromion is a fluid-filled sac called the bursa. The bursa provides lubrication and cushions the tendons from bone. Another shoulder joint called the acromioclavicular joint, or AC joint, acts as a hinge for raising the shoulder.

In sports where arms are raised over the head, such as baseball, volleyball, badminton, tennis or swimming, rotator cuff injuries are frequent. With the arms elevated above a line parallel to the ground, these muscles become stressed and stretched out, loosening the head of the joint within the shoulder socket resulting in shoulder impingement.

Unfortunately, untreated impingements can shorten the career of the most talented athlete. A torn rotator cuff muscle can end it. A proper exercise program will strengthen the rotator cuff muscle so the head of the shoulder will not slip out of the socket and will eliminate inflammation and irritation.

Simple wear and tear produces some of the most common shoulder problems, such as bursitis, inflammation of the bursa, or tendonitis, inflammation in the bicep's tendons or rotator cuff. Although both are quite painful, the pain of tendonitis is present along the length of the tendon only when using the tender body part. Bursitis pain is constant and isolated to one specific spot.

Other rotator cuff ailments related to wear and tear include tears, calcium deposits and arthritis, but they are also caused by muscle imbalance and overuse. Like any other body area, shoulder muscles are subject to pulls caused by overcontraction or overstretching.

Common shoulder problems not associated with wear or degeneration include sprains, ligament tears, dislocations and fractures. Treatment for shoulder problems range from rest, ice, massage, stretching, strengthening, and medication to surgery.

Shoulder Pain And Rotator Cuff
General Massage Areas

Maximum
Pressure

35 LBS
25 LBS

Moderate
Pressure

25 LBS
15 LBS

Minimum
Pressure

15 LBS
5 LBS

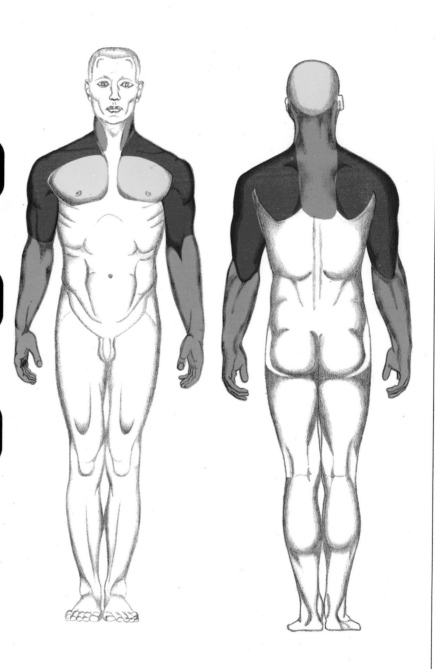

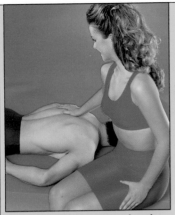

Use palm technique to relax the shoulder and scapula (shoulder blade).

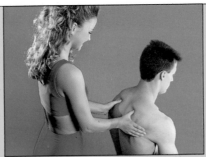

Move thumbs in a circular motion up and down between the shoulder blades.

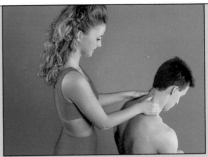

Head forward, apply thumb technique of both hands along the muscles of the neck.

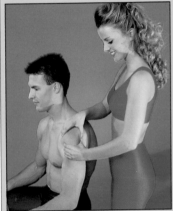

Use both hands to knead Receiver's shoulder.

TRIGGER POINTS

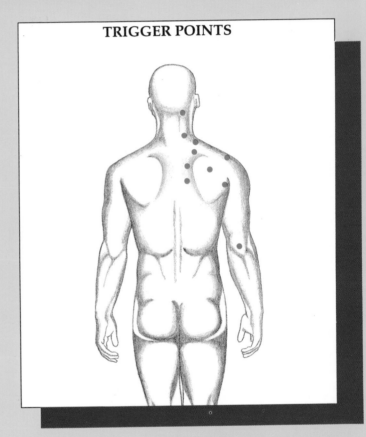

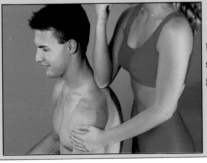

Use knuckle technique to massage the muscles above and around the shoulder blade.

Use elbow technique on the shoulder muscles and trigger points.

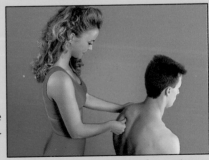

Use thumb technique to work on trigger points along the shoulder blade.

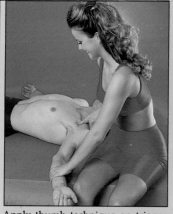

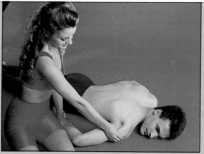

Use thumb to work on trigger points along the shoulder and scapula.

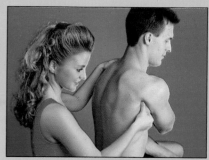

Use thumb technique on trigger points around Receiver's arm pit.

Apply thumb technique on trigger points of the deltoid and pectoral muscles.

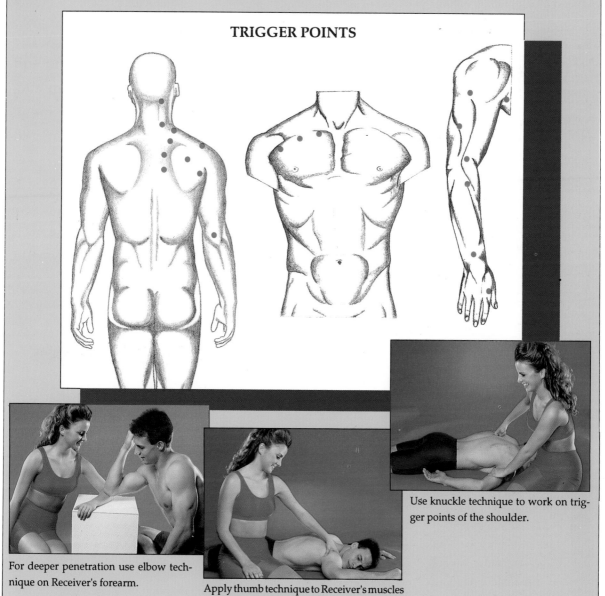

TRIGGER POINTS

For deeper penetration use elbow technique on Receiver's forearm.

Apply thumb technique to Receiver's muscles around the arm pit.

Use knuckle technique to work on trigger points of the shoulder.

SHOULDER / ROTATOR CUFF
S T R E T C H I N G

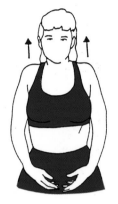

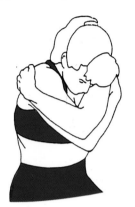

SHOULDER SHRUG ROTATION

Standing with arms at sides as shown, shrug shoulders as high as possible and hold for three seconds. Then pull shoulders back, pushing shoulder blades inward, and hold three seconds. Relax and repeat 10 times.

RHOMBOID STRETCH

Wrap arms around chest and grab shoulder blades as shown. With mouth close, bring chin to chest and try to pull shoulder blades forward until slight stretch is felt. Hold 10 to 20 seconds. Repeat 3 times.

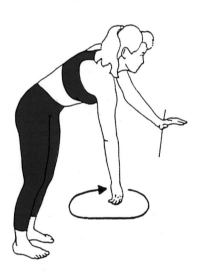

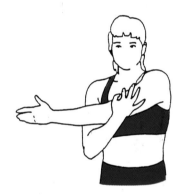

INFERIOR CUFF STRETCH

Stand as shown, grasp arm just above elbow and gently pull elbow toward body. Hold 10 to 20 seconds. Repeat 3 times with each arm.

PENDULAR EXERCISE

Stand with body bent forward as shown, knees slightly bent, one hand resting on bar or table, the other arm hanging limp. (a) Make small clockwise circles with extended arm, gradually increasing in size. Make 10 circles. (b) In same manner, make 10 counter-clockwise circles. (c) Then swing arm forward-backward arcs 10 times, and (d) swing arm side to side in front of body 10 times. Keep shoulder relaxed and use body motion to swing arm.

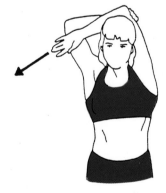

POSTERIOR CUFF STRETCH

Standing as shown, raise arm over head and grasp arm near elbow. Pull arm toward body until gentle stretch is felt and hold 20 seconds. Repeat 3 times with each arm.

SHOULDER / ROTATOR CUFF
S   T   R   E   T   C   H   I   N   G

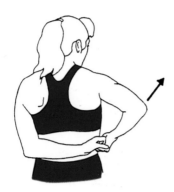

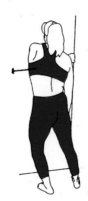

SUPRASPINATUS STRETCH
Standing as shown, position arm behind back and clasp hands together. Pull arm forward until gentle stretch is felt and hold 20 seconds. Repeat 3 times with each arm.

RHOMBOID STRETCH
Stand at wall or doorway as shown, arm across chest, hand grasping corner, knee slightly bent. Shift weight and lean to side, until gentle stretch is felt in shoulder. Hold 20 seconds. Repeat 3 times with each arm.

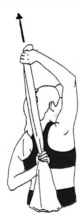

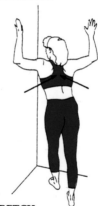

TOWEL STRETCH
Holding towel behind back as shown, pull on towel, raising lower arm as high as possible without discomfort. Hold 5 to 10 seconds and slowly release. Then switch arms and pull on towel and bring the top arm down as far as possible without discomfort. Hold 5 to 10 seconds. Repeat 3 times each way.

PECTORALIS STRETCH
Stand in corner with hands at shoulder level as shown. Lean forward until stretch is felt across chest. Hold 20 seconds. Repeat 3 times.

SHOULDER / ROTATOR CUFF
S T R E N G T H E N I N G

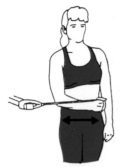

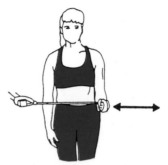

INTERNAL ROTATION-Thera-band

Attach band waist high to bar or doorknob. Standing as shown, arm against side, elbow bent at 90 degree angle, grasp band and pull across body toward opposite arm. Hold 5 seconds then slowly return to starting position. Repeat 10 times. Do 3 sets of 10 repetitions.

EXTERNAL ROTATION-Thera-band

Attach band waist high to bar or doorknob. Standing as shown, arm against side, elbow bent at 90 degree angle, grasp band and pull across body. Hold 5 seconds then slowly return to starting position. Repeat 10 times. Do 3 sets of 10 repetitions.

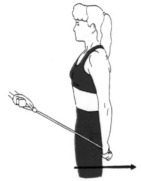

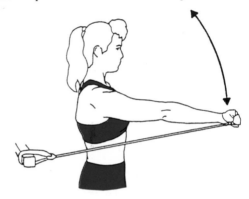

EXTENSION ROTATION-Thera-band

Attach band waist high to bar or doorknob. Stand facing bar as shown, arm at side, elbow straight. Grasp band and pull straight back. Hold 5 seconds then slowly return to starting position. Repeat 10 times. Do 3 sets of 10 repetitions.

FLEXION-Thera-band

Attach band waist high to bar doorknob. Stand back to bar as shown, arm at side. Keep elbow straight and pull band out then up. Hold 5 seconds then slowly return to starting position. Repeat 10 times. Do 3 sets of 10 repetitions.

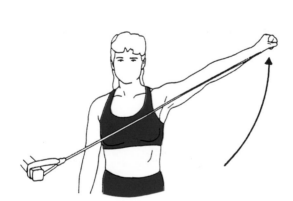

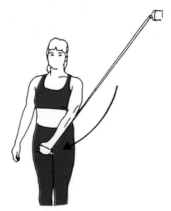

ABDUCTION-Thera-band

Attach band waist high to bar or doorknob. Standing as shown, keep elbow straight and pull band straight up from side. Hold 5 seconds then slowly return to starting position. Repeat 10 times. Do 3 sets of 10 repetitions.

ADDUCTION-Thera-band

Attach band overhead to bar or pole. Standing as shown, grasp band above and pull diagonally down across body. Hold 5 seconds then slowly return to starting position. Repeat 10 times. Do 3 sets of 10 repetitions.

SHOULDER / ROTATOR CUFF
S T R E N G T H E N I N G

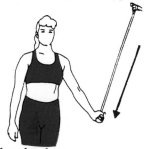

DIAGONALS -Thera-band

Attach band overhead to bar or pole. Standing as shown, grasp band above, palm to back, pull band down and across the body, rotating arm. Return slowly. Repeat 10 times. Do 3 sets of 10 repetitions.

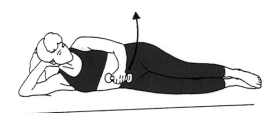

EXTERNAL ROTATION

Lie on side as shown, head supported by hand, knees slightly bent. With weight in hand as shown, bend elbow to 90 degree angle and slowly lift weight until forearm is parallel to floor, then slowly lower. Keep elbow supported at side, palm down. Return slowly. Repeat 10 times. Do 3 sets of 10 repetitions.

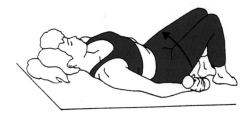

EXTERNAL AND INTERNAL ROTATION

Lie on back as shown, arms to side, elbow bent at 90 degree angle, forearm out. With weight in hand slowly lower forearm to side, then return. Keep elbow supported at side. Repeat 10 times. Do 3 sets of 10 repetitions.

FORWARD PRESS - Thera-band

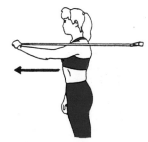

Attach band shoulder height to bar or pole. Standing as shown, grasp band and push forward until arm is straight. Return slowly. Repeat 10 times. Do 3 sets of 10 repetitions.

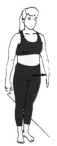

SUPRASPINATUS

Stand with arms at side, weight in each hand, elbows straight. Turn arms so thumbs point to floor, lift arms to side and slightly forward to just below shoulder level. Slowly lower weights and repeat 10 times. Do 3 sets of 10 repetitions.

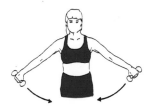

ISOMETRIC SHOULDER ABDUCTION

Standing perpendicular to wall as shown, elbow straight, push against wall with back of hand. Hold 5 seconds, then relax. Repeat 10 times.

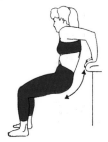

SITTING SHOULDER DEPRESSION

Standing a few inches out from table, feet shoulder width apart, grasp edge as shown and slowly lower body by bending knees until slight stretch is felt. Return slowly. Repeat 10 times.

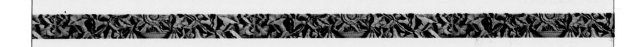

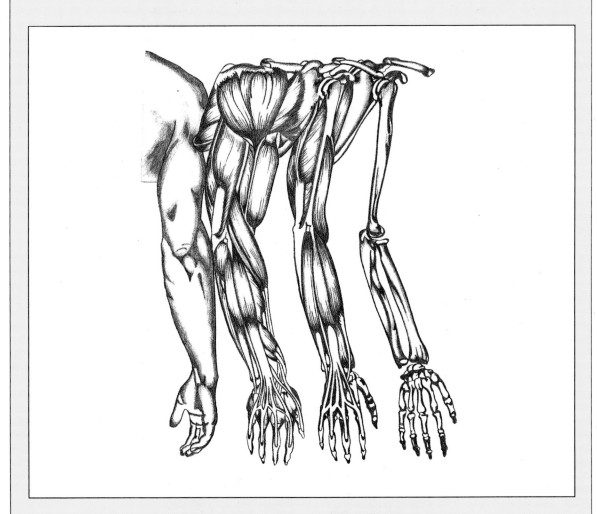

THE ELBOW

The Elbow

The elbow is a joint that permits two separate arm motions—bending and straightening and supination and pronation. Both types of motion are made possible by the joining of three bones. The upper arm bone (humerus) forms the top of the joint and the two forearm bones (radius and ulna) form the bottom. Each forearm bone allows specific movement. The ulna attaches to the upper arm and acts like a hinge for bending and straightening the forearm. The radius fits into the elbow joint and lets the forearm turn for supination and pronation. Ligaments bind the bones together.

Some of the most common elbow problems include sprains, bursitis and tennis elbow. Sprains frequently occur when the ligament that holds the elbow together is partially torn or stretched. Elbow sprains can vary in intensity from mild to severe.

Elbow bursitis is an irritation to the bursa sac, located between skin and bone. Prolonged irritation can lead to swelling causing a buildup of bursa sac fluid. Elbow buritis is easily recognizable and tends to be uncomfortable and awkward. This injury is common in sports in which participants wear no elbow guards or where elbow protection is inadequate.

"Tennis" or golfer's elbow results when there is excessive strain on the forearm muscles. (Most therapist refer to lateral epicondylitis as tennis elbow and medial epicondylitis as golfers elbow). Tennis players and golfers are most frequently affected by this condition as a result of faulty stroke technique. Problems develop when recreational players use wrist movement instead of whole arm and shoulder strokes. Pain develops on the outside of the elbow when the muscles and tendons become inflamed. Pain typically increases during lifting, grasping or rotating hand movement.

"Little League elbow" or "thrower's elbow" is an injury caused by repeated yanking on the elbow's growth center when young pitchers throw too often or too hard. The irritation of the growth center results in an overgrowth of the medial epicondyle. Rehabilitation of this injury includes immobilization and range-of-motion exercises. Unfortunately, the pitcher sometimes loses effectiveness due to this injury.

Another common elbow injury is hyperextended elbow when external forces extend it beyond its normal range. Muscle fibers that hold the elbow joint together tear and cause pain and swelling.

The best way to avoid elbow problems is to rest from the aggreviating motions, to condition muscles properly, and to warm up thoroughly before exercise. Adopt new playing techniques to reduce the force and stress to the forearm muscles and elbow.

Golf And Tennis Elbow
General Massage Areas

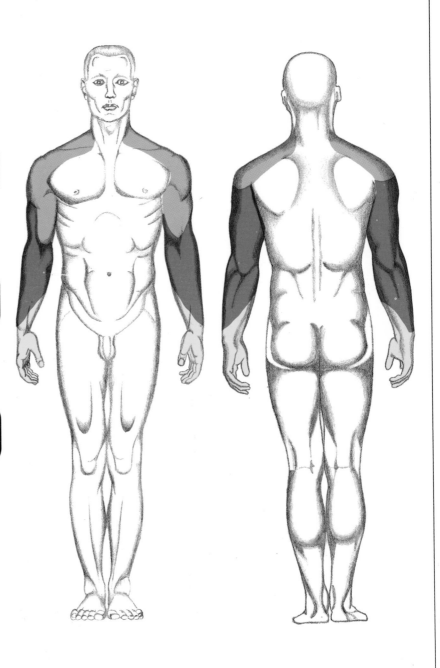

**Maximum
Pressure**

35 LBS
25 LBS

**Moderate
Pressure**

25 LBS
15 LBS

**Minimum
Pressure**

15 LBS
5 LBS

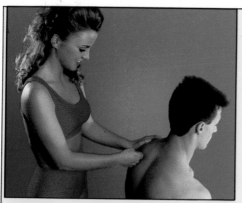

Apply knuckle pressure on trigger points around the shoulder

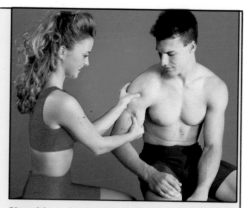

Knead from the shoulder to the elbow using both hands.

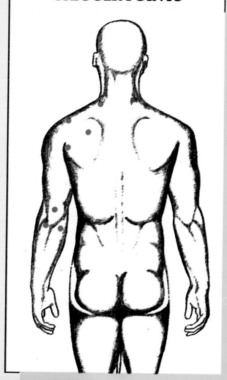

TRIGGER POINTS

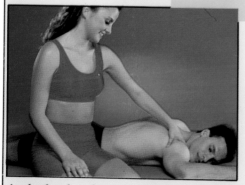

Apply thumb technique to Receiver's muscles around the arm pit.

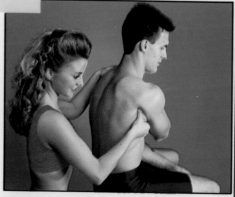

Use thumb technique on trigger points around Receiver's arm pit.

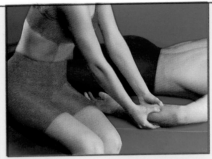

Knead with both hands to relax the forearm
muscles.

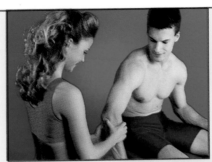

Apply deep circular
pressure with thumbs
on either side of the
elbow.

TRIGGER POINTS

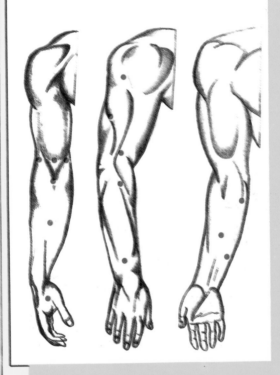

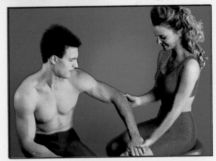

Hold Receiver's hand for stability. Use thumb
technique to trigger points around the elbow
areas.

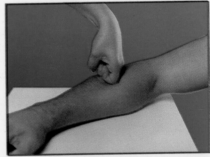

Use knuckles to apply circular pressure across
the muscles of the forearm.

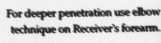

For deeper penetration use elbow
technique on Receiver's forearm.

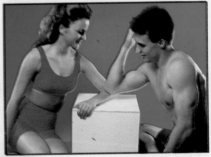

Grasp wrist of Receiver for stability
while using the other hand to knead
the forearm.

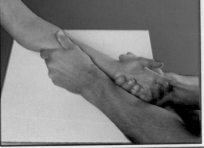

Use knuckle technique on trigger points and
muscles spasms of the forearm.

TRIGGER POINTS

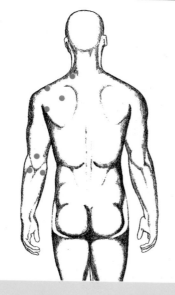
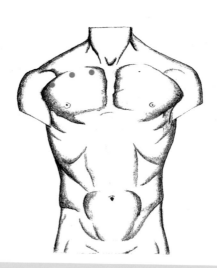

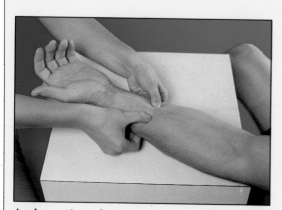

Apply scorpion technique to relieve knots of the forearm.

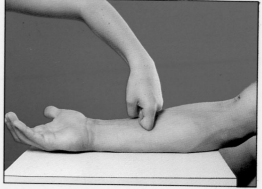

Use knuckle technique to massage spasms and trigger points.

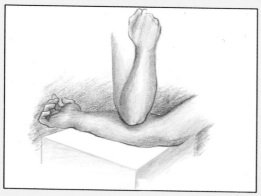

Use elbow technique to massage the muscles of the forearm.

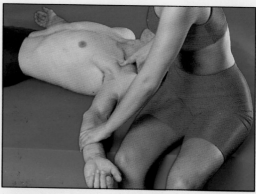

Apply thumb technique on trigger points of the deltoid and pectoral muscles.

ELBOW PAIN
S T R E T C H I N G

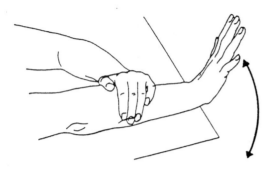

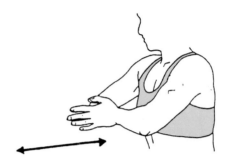

WRIST EXTENSION
With forearm on table, hand and wrist extended over the edge as shown, lift up and down slowly. Repeat 10 times.

WRIST EXTENSION
With arms at shoulder level, elbows straight, palms together, slowly bend elbows, drawing hands in to body as shown. Do not clench hands; keep fingers straight. Repeat 10 times.

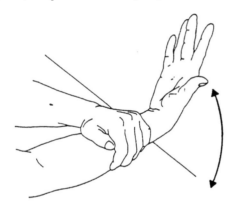

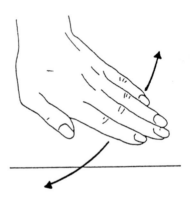

WRIST FLEXION
Rest forearm on table, hand and wrist over edge as shown, palm up. Steady arm with other hand and lift hand up and down slowly. Repeat 10 times.

WRIST DEVIATION
With forearm resting on table, palm down and fingers straight as shown, turn or twist hand toward thumb, then turn or twist to other side. Keep forearm stable with other hand. Repeat 10 times to each side.

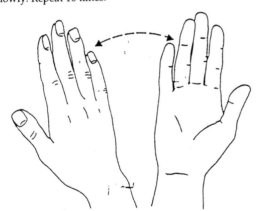

FOREARM PRONATION/SUPINATION
With hands palms up on lap of any flat surface, elbows close to body, turn hands face down, hold 5 seconds, then turn palms up again, hold five seconds. Repeat twenty times.

ELBOW PAIN

S T R E N G T H E N I N G

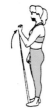

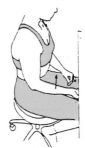

ELBOW FLEXION (THERA-BAND)

Standing with ends of thera - band held in hand and secured under ball of foot, bend elbow and pull hand toward shoulder. Hold five seconds, then slowly lower to starting position. Repeat five times on each hand.

ELBOW FLEXION (ISOMETRIC)

Sitting upright at table as shown, elbow bent 90 degrees, forearm beneath table, push forearm toward table. Hold 5 seconds, then relax. Repeat ten times on each hand.

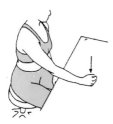

ELBOW EXTENSION (ISOMETRIC)

With forearm resting on table, elbow bent 90 degrees, press forearm down on table. Hold 5 seconds, then relax. Repeat ten times on each hand.

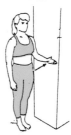

SHOULDER FLEXION (ISOMETRIC)

Standing perpendicular to wall as shown, elbow straight, push arm against wall. Hold 5 seconds, then relax. Repeat ten times on each side.

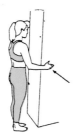

INTERNAL ROTATION (ISOMETRIC)

Standing in door frame or at wall corner, elbow bent 90 degrees, press arm into wall as shown. Hold 5 seconds, then relax. Repeat ten times on each side.

SHOULDER EXTENSION (ISOMETRIC)

Standing with back to wall as shown, push arm back into wall, elbow straight. Hold 5 seconds, then relax. Repeat ten times on each side.

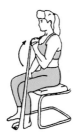

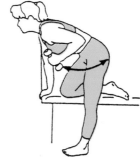

ELBOW FLEXION (THERA-BAND)

Sitting upright on chair or bench as shown, tubing secured under foot and wrapped around fist, curl arm up to chest then lower. Keep elbow close to side, tubing to outside. Repeat ten times on each arm.

TRICEP EXTENSION

Standing at bench as shown, bend elbow, bringing weight to chest. Keep back straight, elbow close to side. Repeat twenty times on each arm.

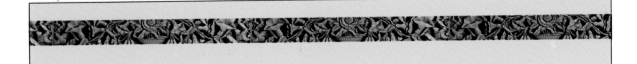

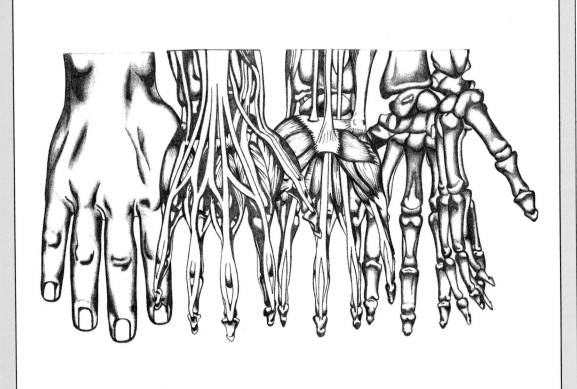

THE WRIST AND HAND

The Wrist and Hand

Eight small bones and several flexible ligaments make up the wrist. The wrist itself lies between the wrist bone and the two forearm bones.

The wrist joint is secured by a flexible sleeve called the capsule, which provides equal movement of the wrist from side to side and up and down. Groups of forearm tendons activate wrist movement in four directions; a separate group controls the fingers and thumb.

Three major nerves of the arm direct all wrist and hand movement. Radial, ulna and median nerves course along the bones in the forearm and into the hand through a canal. The canal is formed by the wrist bones and the transverse carpal ligament.

Connected to the eight wrist bones are five short, strong bones called the metacarpals. Five metacarpal bones form the palm. Thumb mobility depends on a saddle-shaped joint at the base of the thumb and the metacarpal bone.

The four fingers are composed of three bones and the thumb is made up of two bones called phalanges. All phalanges are held together by ligaments and are surrounded by the joint capsule.

The hand, like the wrist, depends on forearm and hand muscles to move. Tendons run across the wrist and into the hand. Intrinsic hand muscles are small and numerous and work with the extrinsic hand muscles to allow gentleness and strength. These same three nerves--radial, median and ulna--which control wrist movement also control all hand muscles and carry messages to and from the brain and skin.

Common wrist and hand problems include sprains, when a wrist, hand or finger is forced into a position which exceeds its normal range of motion; tears, where a ligament or joint capsule is torn or separated from bone; and DeQuervain's tendonitis, inflammation of the two tendons that empower the thumb and allow a 90 degree angle between wrist and thumb.

Basketball players are particularly prone to injuries of wrist and hands. They instinctively extend their hands to stop the momentum of a fall or collision. Unfortunately, the wrist absorbs the impact and a sprain results when the ligaments connecting the carpal bones tear and the bones become partially dislocated.

Finger and hand fractures are common in all games where a ball is volleyed or passed between players. Forcible extension of the fingers, deflection of the ball, and direct blows to the hands can rupture tendons and break the metacarpal bones and phalanges.

"Carpal tunnel syndrome" frequently is an inflammation caused by repeated bending of the wrist such as throwing a baseball or softball. Inflammation of the tendons and tendon sheaths reduces the space in the carpal tunnel compressing the medial nerve resulting in pain, burning and hand numbness. Carpal tunnel syndrome also occurs as a result of normal wear and tear, previous fracture or dislocation, or fluid retention called edema.

Overuse of the wrist or repetitive one-sided movements can cause tendinitis, an inflammation of the thumb tendons attached to the extensor and flexor muscles of the forearm. Tendinitis is common among racquet sportsman, but the likelihood of inflammation can be reduced in training by strengthening the forearm muscles.

Hand and wrist problems are treated with any combination of rest from the aggravating activity, massage, moist heat, ultrasound, injections, medication, splints or surgery.

Wrist And Hand Sprain
General Massage Areas

Maximum Pressure

35 LBS
25 LBS

Moderate Pressure

25 LBS
15 LBS

Minimum Pressure

15 LBS
5 LBS

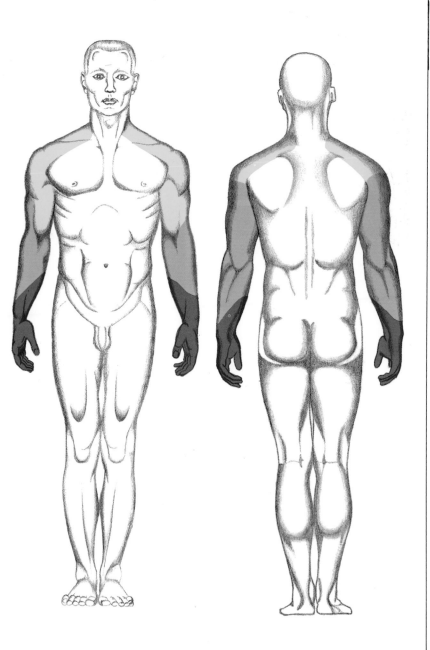

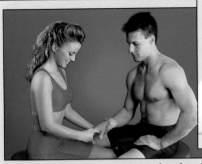

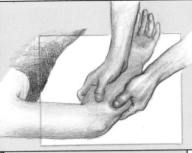

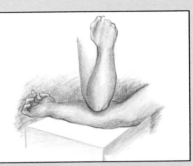

Hold Receiver's forearm in one hand and used the other to gently stretch each finger and the thumb.

Use both hands to knead the forearm.

Use elbow technique to massage the muscles of the forearm.

TRIGGER POINTS

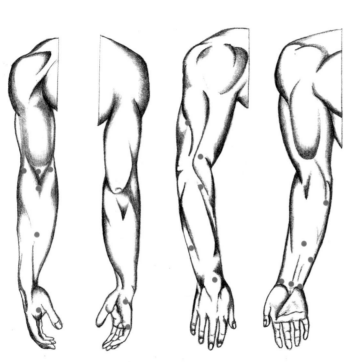

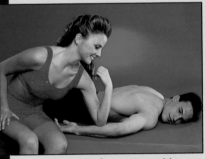

For deeper penetration use elbow technique on Receiver's forearms.

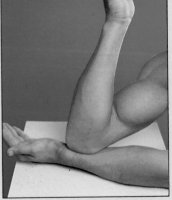

With Receiver in the prone position use elbow technique to massage the forearm.

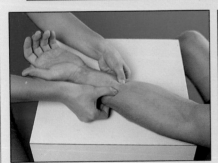

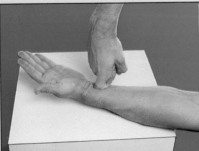

Apply scorpion technique to relieve knots of the forearm.

The knuckle technique may also be used to massage wrist area.

For deeper pressure use the elbow technique.

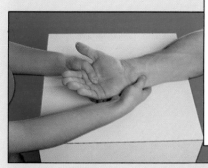

Apply thumb technique to work around the trigger points of the wrist.

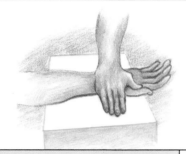

Press your palm in as outward circular motion increase depth gradually.

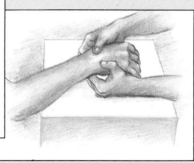

Use thumb to apply alternating pressure to the trigger point areas of the wrist and hand.

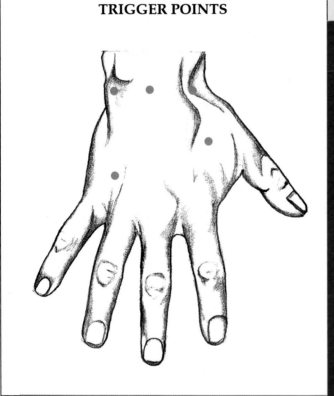

TRIGGER POINTS

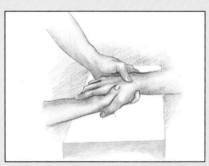

Apply thumb technique on both hands of Receiver's wrist.

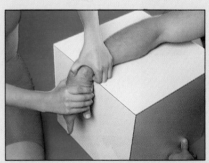

Use thumb technique on Receiver's stretched wrist.

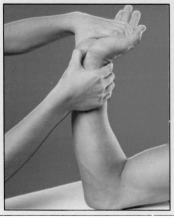

Apply thumb pressure on Receiver's stretched wrist, work on the trigger points.

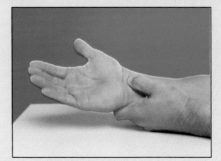

Use own hand to knead the wrist.

WRIST AND HAND
S   T   R   E   T   C   H   I   N   G

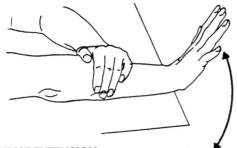

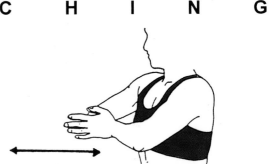

WRIST EXTENSION

With forearm on table, hand and wrist extended over the edge as shown, lift up and down slowly. Repeat 10 times.

WRIST EXTENSION

With arms at shoulder level, elbows straight, palms together, slowly bend elbows, drawing hands in to body as shown. Do not clench hands; keep fingers straight. Repeat 10 times.

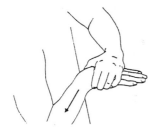

BENDING WRIST DOWN

Place hand on table, wrist down with other hand on top to hold it flat. Bend forearm down as shown. Hold the stretch 10 to 20 seconds then return to starting position. Repeat 3 times.

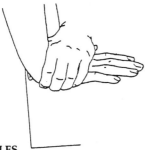

WRIST CIRCLES

With palm down on table, the other hand on top to hold it flat, move arm in small circles then gradually increase to larger circles. Repeat in reverse direction.

BENDING WRIST UP

Place arm on table, palm down, the other hand on top to hold it flat. Raise elbow and forearm slowly off table, bending bottom hand at the wrist as shown. Hold the stretch 10 to 20 seconds then return to starting position. Repeat 3 times.

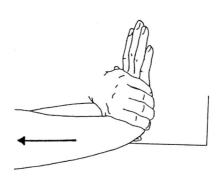

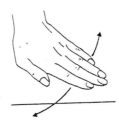

WRIST DEVIATION

With forearm resting on table, palm down and fingers straight as shown, turn or twist hand toward thumb, then turn or twist to other side. Keep forearm stable with other hand. Repeat 10 times.

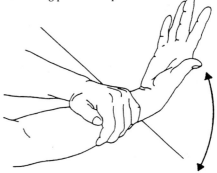

WRIST FLEXION

Rest forearm on table, hand and wrist over edge as shown, palm up. Steady arm with other hand and lift hand up and down slowly. Repeat 10 times.

WRIST AND HAND
S T R E N G T H E N I N G

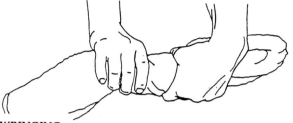

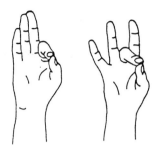

WRINGING
Hold terry cloth towel in hands and "wring out" as shown. Bend one wrist down, the other wrist up. Repeat wringing in opposite direction. Repeat 10 times each way.

FINGER PRESS
Press thumb to each finger, beginning with forefinger, working toward pinkie, then reverse. Repeat 10 times.

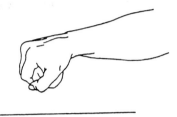

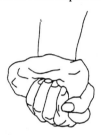

THERA-PUTTY EXERCISE
With thera-putty in hand, palm down, as shown, press and squeeze putty with thumb and fingers. Repeat 10 times. Do 3 sets of 10 repetitions.

THERA-PUTTY EXERCISE
With thera-putty in palm of hand, push each finger into it one at a time as shown. Repeat 10 times. Do 3 sets of 10 repetitions.

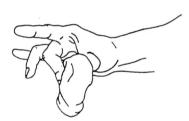

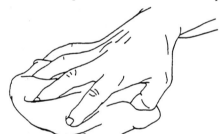

THERA-PUTTY EXERCISE
With thera-putty between thumb and each finger one at a time. Repeat 10 times with each finger. Do 3 sets of 10 repetitions.

THERA-PUTTY EXERCISE
With thera-putty on table, curl finger then push putty outward. Repeat 10 times. Do 3 sets of 10 repetitions.

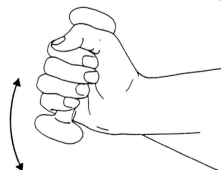

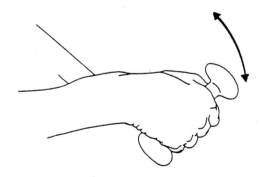

WRIST EXERCISE-WITH WEIGHTS
With forearm resting on edge of table, hand holding weight off edge, thumb up as shown, raise and lower weight. Repeat 10 times. Do 3 sets of 10 repetitions.

WRIST EXERCISE-WITH WEIGHTS
With forearm resting on edge of table, hand holding weight off edge, thumb down as shown, raise and lower weight. Repeat 10 times. Do 3 sets of 10 repetitions.

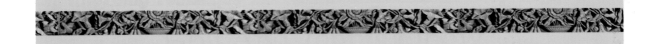

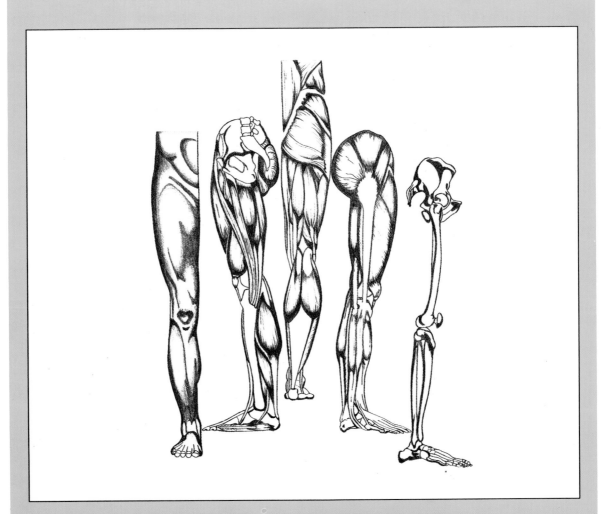

THE THIGHS
(HAMSTRING PULL & QUADRICEPS PULL)

The Thigh
Hamstring Pull/Groin, Hip Flexor and Quadriceps Pull

The hamstring muscles are located in the back of the thighs. Their function is to pull or bend the knee and extend the hips. The hamstring originates in the pelvis and is protected by the buttocks. Two of the hamstring muscles descend down the inner part of the thigh and attach to the inner part of the tibia (lower leg bone). The other hamstring muscle descends down the outer thigh and attaches to the fibula (small outer leg bone).

Probably the most common injury in the thigh and the most common muscle pull is the hamstring pull. The hamstrings can rip or pull when the body is tight and unyielding before exercise. These muscle pulls are usually the result of overstretching, not overcontracting. Hamstring pulls occur when the hamstring resists the opposing muscle, the quadricep. Initial treatment of hamstring pulls involved ice, compression and rest. Gentle stretching exercises should be started as early as the second day following injury while the muscle is still recuperating. Warming up sufficiently and continued stretching are the best ways to prevent hamstring problems.

The quadricep muscle is the large muscle in the front thigh which straightens the knee and flexes the hip. The quad moves opposite the hamstring, and is generally stronger. Pulls or tears in the quadricep muscle are less common than hamstring pulls, but the quadricep muscle will sometimes pull during running or jumping activities.

More often, a blow to the contracted quadriceps muscle during contact sports will crush muscle fibers against the femur bone causing rupture. If this happens, ice should be applied with the knee bent as far as possible to compress the quadricep muscle and to stop possible muscle bleeding. This treatment should be followed by stretching and flexing exercises.

Hamstring Pull
General Massage Areas

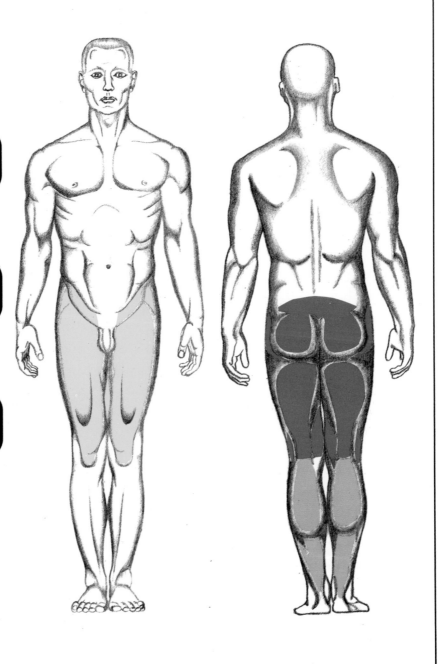

Maximum Pressure

35 LBS
25 LBS

Moderate Pressure

25 LBS
15 LBS

Minimum Pressure

15 LBS
5 LBS

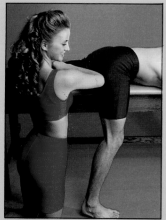

In this stretched position, for maximum release, use elbow technique on Receiver's hamstring.

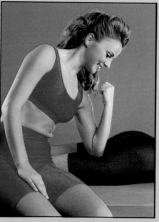

Use elbow technique for deeper penetration onto the Receiver's hamstring.

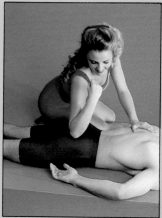

To effectively break down scar tissue of the bulky hamstring muscles use the elbow technique with the aid of bodyweight.

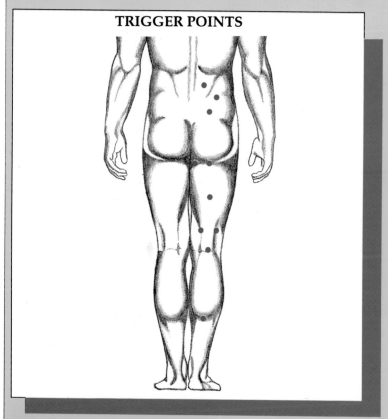

TRIGGER POINTS

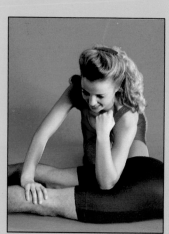

Use the elbow technique to work on trigger points and spasm around the hips and buttocks.

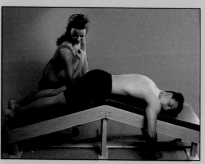

Use elbow technique on Receiver's hamstring.

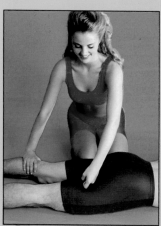

The knuckle technique can also be used to break down scar tissue.

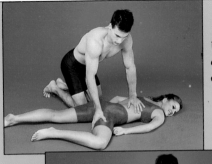

Use thumb technique to apply deep circular pressure on trigger points on ilio-tibial band.

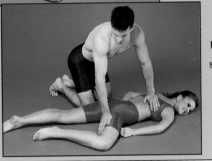

Use palm technique to relax hamstring and ilio-tibial band.

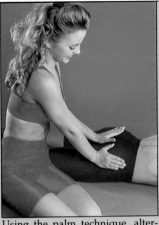

Using the palm technique, alternate pressure between the hands to massage the hips and buttock muscles.

TRIGGER POINTS

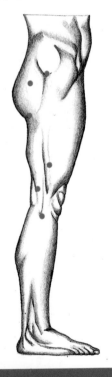

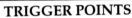

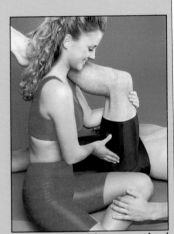

Rest the Receiver's leg on your shoulder. Use thumb technique to massage the hamstring trigger points.

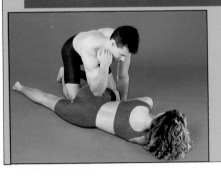

Receiver on side and leg bent. Use elbow to work on spasms around piriformis muscles and sacro-iliac joint.

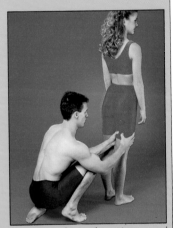

For convenience, in a stance position use thumb technique on Receiver's hamstring.

HAMSTRING

S T R E T C H I N G

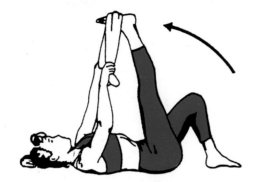

HAMSTRING STRETCH (WITH TOWEL)

Lying on floor, one knee bent as shown, loop towel around other foot. Tighten stomach muscles and raise leg up until slight tightness is felt. Keep knee joint locked and pull towards the head. Repeat three times with each leg.

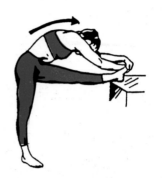

ATHLETIC HAMSTRING STRETCH (TABLE)

Stand erect with heel on counter or barre about hip height. Slowly roll upper body forward; place hands on foot, calf, or thigh. Hold stretch 20 seconds. Repeat three times with each leg.

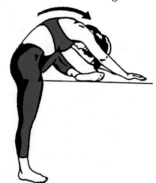

PIRIFORMIS STRETCH

Position body with one leg bent on counter or barre as shown. Curl upper body over bent leg and reach arms forward. Hold, then repeat three times with each leg.

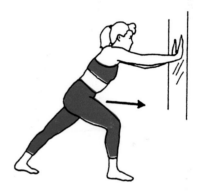

CALF STRETCH

Standing at wall with one foot back 3-4 feet from wall, opposite knee bent, lean against wall with hands. Lower hips until stretch is felt. Hold for 20 seconds, then repeat three times on each leg. Keep back leg straight, heels flat.

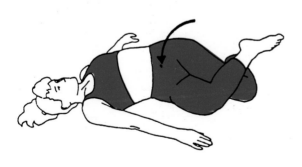

ATHLETIC TRUNK ROLL

Lie on back with knees bent. Cross one leg over the other, rotate hips, and push the lower knee to the floor. Hold 10 seconds, then repeat three times on each side. Keep shoulders and hands flat against the floor.

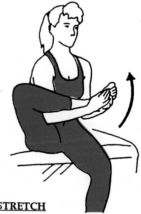

SITTING YOGA STRETCH

Sit erect on chair or bench, one leg crossed the other. Cradle bent leg in arms and pull upward toward chest, keeping back straight. Hold stretch for 10 seconds, then repeat three times on each side.

HAMSTRING
S T R E N G T H E N I N G

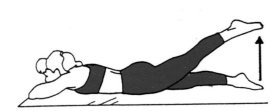

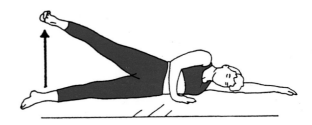

HIP EXTENSION
Lying on stomach as shown, legs straight, lift leg up. Keep knee straight, hold for 10 seconds, then return to starting position. Repeat five times on each leg.

SIDE-LYING HIP ABDUCTION
Lying on side as shown, arm overhead, tighten front thigh muscle and lift leg 8-10 inches from floor. Repeat ten times on each side.

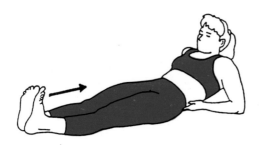

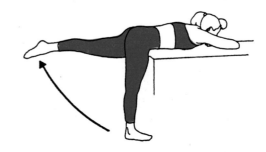

HAMSTRING SET
Lying on floor as shown, arms supporting upper body, flex muscle on back of thigh by pulling heel back with knee slightly bent. Hold 5 seconds, relax and repeat ten times.

SINGLE LEG LIFT
With upper body resting on table, legs off edge as shown, lift one leg as high as possible. Hold for 5 seconds. Repeat five times on each leg.

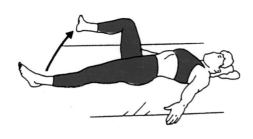

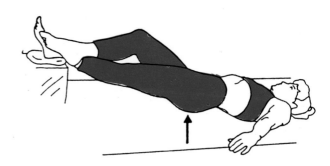

HIP AND KNEE FLEXION
Lying on back as shown, legs straight, lift leg, bending at knee and hip toward outside. Bring knee toward chest as far as possible. Keep other leg straight and flat. Repeat ten times on each leg.

HIP EXTENSION
With heel on 6" box or step, cross ankles as shown. With body extended, raise right gluteus off floor to full hip extension. Hold 3-5 seconds, then relax. Repeat five times on each leg.

Quadriceps Pull, Groin, Hip Flexor
General Massage Areas

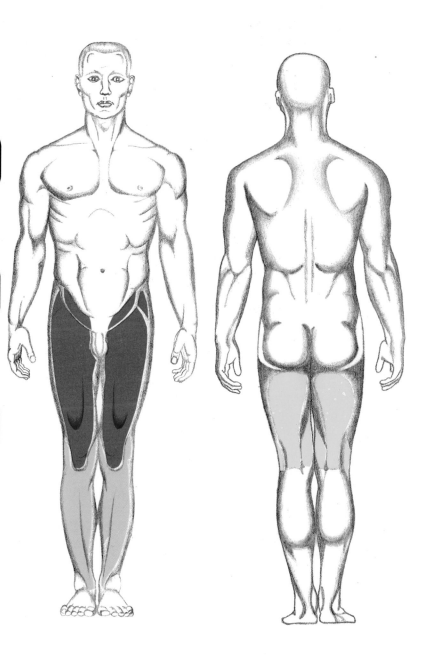

Maximum Pressure

35 LBS
25 LBS

Moderate Pressure

25 LBS
15 LBS

Minimum Pressure

15 LBS
5 LBS

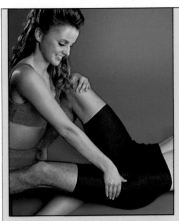

Use thumb technique to work on Receiver's hip flexor.

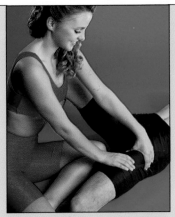

Use both hands to knead Receiver's quadriceps.

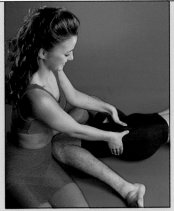

Use both thumbs to massage the hip flexor and quadriceps.

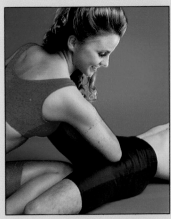

Use elbow technique on stretched hip flexor muscles.

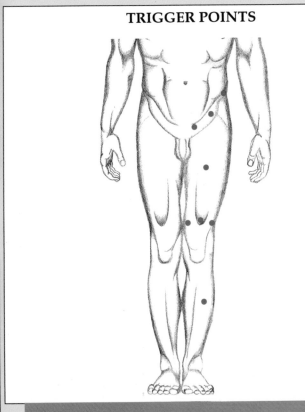

TRIGGER POINTS

Use scorpion technique on Receiver's hip flexor.

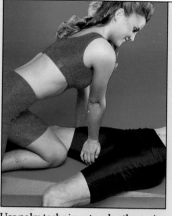

Use palm technique to relax the groin muscles while Receiver's in stretch position.

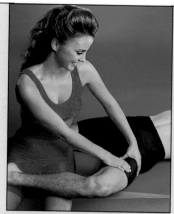

Knead the stretched Quadriceps and groin muscles.

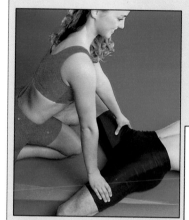

Apply thumb technique on Receiver's stretched groin muscles.

TRIGGER POINTS

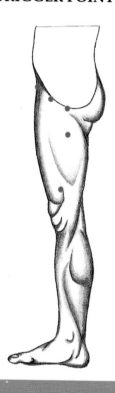

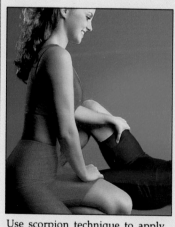

Use scorpion technique to apply circular motion pressure down the quadriceps muscles.

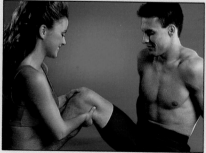

Use thumb technique to massage the trigger points and spasms.

QUADRICEPS

S T R E T C H I N G

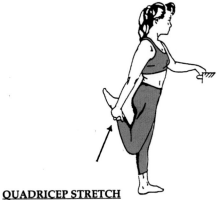

QUADRICEP STRETCH
Standing at barre or counter, grasp ankle with hand as shown. Pull up slowly toward buttocks. Push pelvis forward to increase stretch. Hold 20 seconds. Repeat three times on each leg.

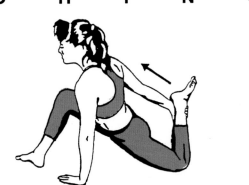

THE ATHLETIC QUAD STRETCH
Kneel on one knee, front leg at 90 degree angle as shown. With right hand grasp left foot, slowly lower front hip toward floor while gently pulling ankle toward buttocks. Hold 20 seconds. Repeat three times on each side.

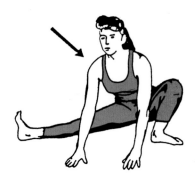

ATHLETIC GROIN STRETCH
Squat with one leg bent, one leg extended, arms forward as shown. Slowly lower hips toward floor. Hold stretch, then switch sides. Do not bounce. Use hands for stability. Repeat three times on each side.

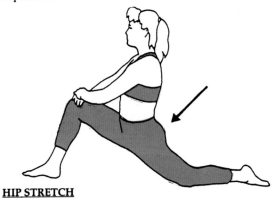

HIP STRETCH
Kneel on floor with front knee bent at 90 degree angle and back leg extended. Tighten stomach muslces and shift weight forward on front foot. Hold stretch 20 seconds, then repeat three times on each side.

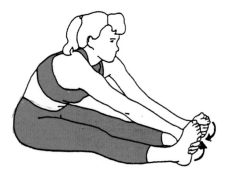

SHIN STRETCH
Sitting as shown, legs straight, rotate ankles to return feet inward. Grab feet with hands at the arch and gently pull towards body. Hold stretch for 20 seconds. Relax and then repeat five times.

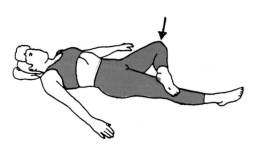

THE HIP TURN
Lying on back as shown, cross ankle over opposite leg just above the knee. Let bent knee slowly fall outward. Use muscles to stretch and hold for ten seconds. Return to starting position and repeat on other side.

QUADRICEPS

S T R E N G T H E N I N G

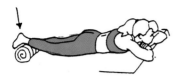

QUAD SET WITH KNEE BENT

Lying on stomach with bolster or rolled towel under ankle as shown, push ankle down into bolster until leg is as straight as possible. Repeat five times on each side.

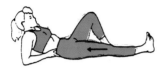

QUAD SET

Resting on forearms, one knee bent as shown, tighten front thigh muscles of extended leg to pull knee cap toward body, lift leg 6-8 inches from floor. Hold for 10 seconds. Repeat five times on each leg.

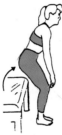

SIT TO STAND

Sit on edge of chair as shown. Lean forward, stand up and get balance. Then sit back down slowly, keeping feet in same position. Use hip and knee muscles, not hands. Repeat five times.

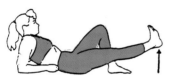

STRAIGHT LEG RAISE

Resting on forearms, one knee bent as shown, tighten muscles on front and back of thighs, lock knee, and lift leg 8-10 inches from floor. Hold for 10 seconds, relax and repeat five times on each side.

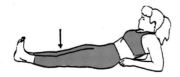

QUADRICEPS SET

Resting on forearms as shown, tighten front thigh muscles by pushing knees down so leg is straight as possible. Hold 5 seconds. Repeat five times.

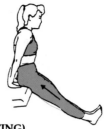

QUAD SET (SITTING)

Sitting on edge of chair with legs outstretched, knees straight as shown, flex front thigh muscles, pulling knee caps toward body. Hold for 10 seconds. Repeat five times on each leg.

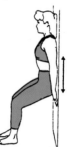

WALL SQUATS

Stand with back and shoulders against wall, feet about eight inches out and knees slightly bent, as shown. Slowly slide down wall and hold about halfway to a sitting position. Slide back up wall and repeat five times.

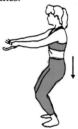

SEMI SQUAT

Holding onto bar or counter as shown, bend knees slowly and hold about halfway to a sitting position. Come up slowly, relax and repeat five times. Do not put pressure or stress on knees. Use thigh muscles and keep back straight.

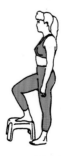

STEP UPS

Standing at side of 6-8" step, position foot on step as shown. Step up then down. Repeat twenty times.

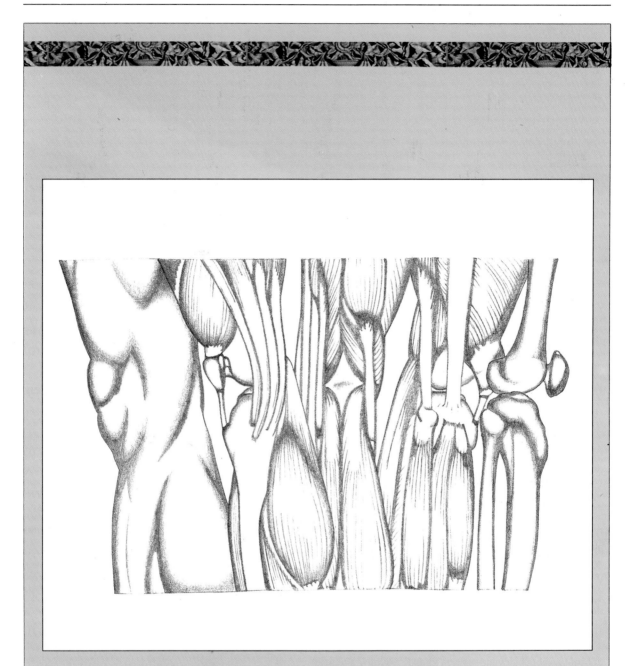

THE KNEE

The Knee

The knee is a large complex joint that bends the leg and joins the femur and tibia (upper and lower leg bones). Articular cartilage covers the end of the leg bones and the underside of the kneecap, enabling them to act as one smooth hinge. Ligaments hold the bones together.

Four large muscles on the front of the thigh, called quadriceps, help the knee to extend. The kneecap is located within the quadriceps tendon which inserts into the tibia just below the kneecap, where the prepatellar bursa exists.

Cartilage, such as the meniscus, absorbs joint shock. Anterior cartilage helps cushion and align the bones. Fibrous sacs of fluid reduce friction between knee bones, ligaments and tendons. A healthy knee allows bones to glide on the cartilages smoothly, while ligaments, tendons and muscles keep the joint aligned, strong and flexible. The knee has two major ligament systems, five capsule ligaments and two additional ligaments called anterior and posterior cruciate which help to stabilize the knee.

The frequently irritated muscles are those on the inside of the knee, such as the hamstrings abductors which come together to form the pes anserinus as they insert into the tibia.

A knee injury is the most common joint injury accounting for one-forth of all injuries and the most likely injury to end an athlete's career. There are five common areas where injuries occur: Ligaments, cartilages, knee muscles, kneecap, and tendons.

"Runner's knee" or "walker's knee," known medically as chondromalacia patella, is the most common overuse injury to the knee. Misalignment of the kneecap in its groove causes friction and erodes the cartilage on the side of the groove and at the back of the kneecap. The source of the problem is not the knee but over-pronation of the feet which turns the knees inward. Over-pronation of the feet can be corrected with an orthotic devices fitted inside the shoe to keep the feet and knees properly aligned.

Another common complaint of runners is iliotibial band syndrome resulting in progressive pain beginning 10 to 20 minutes into a run. The cause is a tight iliotibial band, the hard fiber at the outside of the thigh extending down to the knee. Sometimes the band is overdeveloped and tightened with exercise and treatment and cure involves simple stretching moves.

Other common knee injuries include ligament sprain, Osgood Schlatter's Diease, dislocated patella, bursitis, osteoarthritis and rheumatoid arthritis.

Ligament sprains or tears occur when one of the seven knee ligaments is ripped or torn. These sprains vary in degrees of severity but usually exhibit knee instability as a symptom.

Osgood Schlatter's Disease results from bone changes which cause an inflammed bump to appear below the kneecap. A dislocated patella occurs when the knee is not properly aligned and tends to pop out of place. Chrondomalacia is an erosion of articular cartilage.

Bursitis is an irritation of the bursa, and its symptoms include tenderness, increase in local temperature, swelling and loss of mobility.

Osteoarthritis, a result of agin is a gradual breakdown of articular cartilage that leads to joint deformity. Symptoms include aches, pain, stiffness, swelling, and grinding.

Rheumatoid arthritis, although not a direct result of the aging process, is an inflammation and thickening of the synovial lining of joints. This condition sometimes deteriorates to the point of deformity. Symptoms include pain, stiffness, increase in local temperature, and joint swelling.

Strong knees require strong leg muscles conditioned through exercise. Begin slowly with gentle knee exercises to build strength, but do not aggravate an existing problem. When adequate leg strength is acquired, gradually intensify the exercise program.

Runner's Knee
General Massage Areas

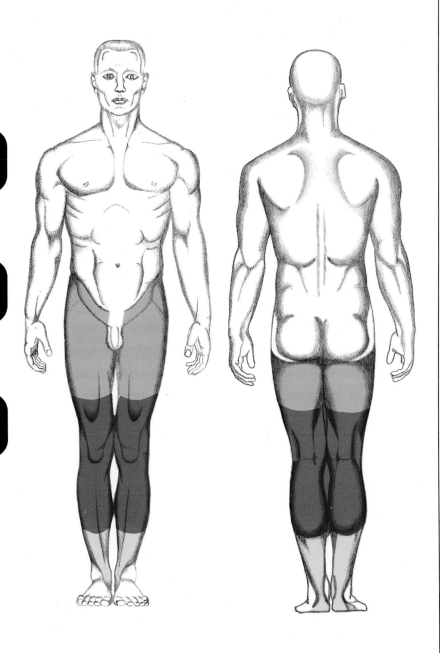

Maximum
Pressure

35 LBS
25 LBS

Moderate
Pressure

25 LBS
15 LBS

Minimum
Pressure

15 LBS
5 LBS

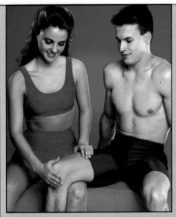

Move palm in a circular motion to relax tightness around the knee.

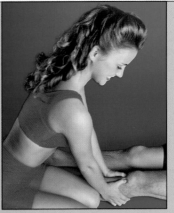

Use both hands to knead around the knee cap.

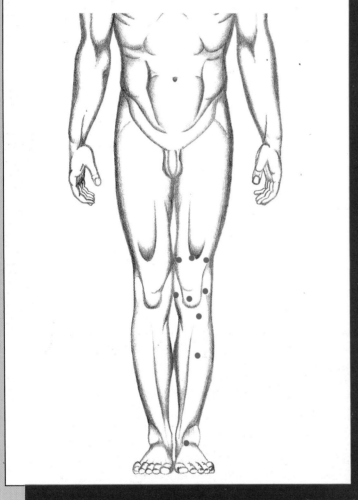

TRIGGER POINTS

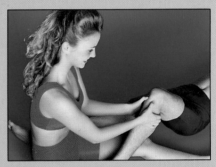

Use both thumbs on trigger points around the knee cap.

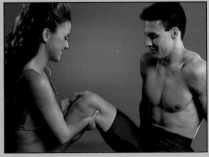

Use scorpion technique to apply circular motion pressure up and down the quadriceps muscles.

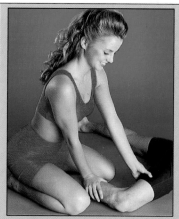

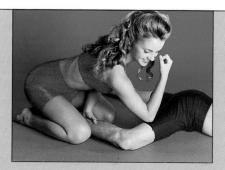

Use elbow technique on Receiver's ilio-tibial band. (I.T. Band) Trigger points.

Use thumb technique to work on ilio-tibial band spasms and trigger points.

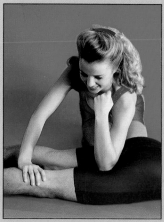

Use the elbow technique to work on trigger points and spasm around the hips and buttocks.

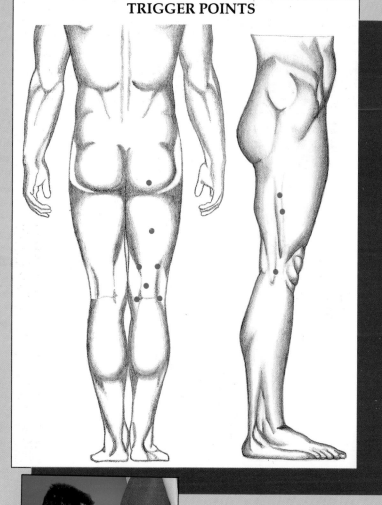

TRIGGER POINTS

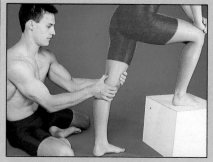

While Receiver is stretching the calf and hamstring, manipulate trigger points around the back of the knee.

Use both thumbs to work on trigger points around and behind the knee.

KNEE PROBLEM
S T R E T C H I N G

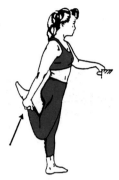

QUADRICEP STRETCH
Standing at barre or counter, grasp ankle with hand as shown. Pull up slowly toward buttocks. Push pelvis forward to increase stretch. Hold 20 seconds. Repeat three times on each leg.

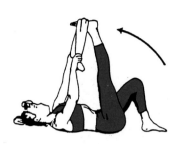

HAMSTRING STRETCH (WITH TOWEL)
Lying on floor, one knee bent as shown, loop towel around other foot. Tighten stomach muscles and raise leg up until slight tightness is felt. Keep knee joint locked and pull towards the head. Repeat three times with each leg.

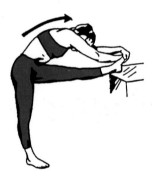

ATHLETIC HAMSTRING STRETCH (TABLE)
Stand erect with heel on counter or barre about hip height. Slowly roll upper body forward; place hands on foot, calf, or thigh. Hold stretch 20 seconds. Repeat three times on each leg.

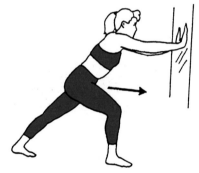

CALF STRETCH
Standing at wall with one foot back 3-4 feet from wall, opposite knee bent, lean against wall with hands. Lower hips until stretch is felt. Hold for 20 seconds, then repeat three times on each leg. Keep back leg straight, heels flat.

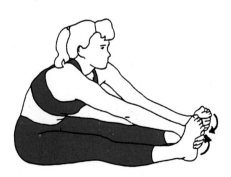

SHIN STRETCH
Sitting as shown, legs straight, rotate ankles to return feet inward. Grab feet with hands at the arch and gently pull towards body. Hold stretch for 20 seconds. Relax and then repeat five times.

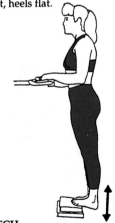

HEEL CORD STRETCH
With balls of feet on book or step, weight forward, hands grasping barre or counter, lower heels toward floor. Hold, then return to starting position. Do not bounce. Repeat 5 times.

KNEE PROBLEM
S T R E N G T H E N I N G

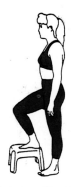

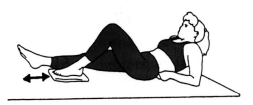

STEP UPS
Standing at side of 6-8" step, position foot on step as shown. Step up then down. Repeat twenty times.

HEEL SLIDE
Lying on floor as shown, flex knee and place a towel under the heel pull heel toward buttocks. Hold, then slide heel away to straighten leg. Repeat 3 times on each leg.

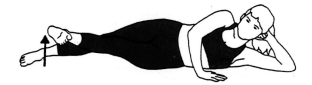

HIP ABDUCTION
Lying on side as shown, tighten front thigh muscle and lift lower leg 8-10 inches from floor. Hold for 10 seconds. Lower slowly. Repeat 5 times on each side.

TERMINAL KNEE EXTENSION
Lying on back, place bolster under knees as shown. Lift foot up until leg is straight, knee supported by bolster. Hold, then slowly lower to starting position. Repeat 5 times on each side.

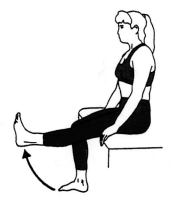

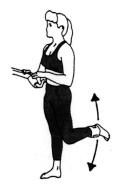

FULL ARC QUADS
Sitting upright in chair or on edge of table or bed as shown, extend leg until knee is straight. Hold for 10 seconds then lower leg to starting position. Repeat 5 times on each side.

HAMSTRING CURL (STANDING WITH WEIGHTS)
Standing up, hands holding barre or counter, cuff weight secured to ankle as shown, bend knee and raise heel toward buttocks. Slowly lower to starting position. Repeat 10 times.

KNEE PROBLEM
S T R E N G T H E N I N G

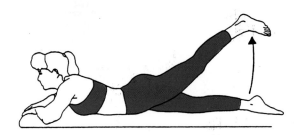

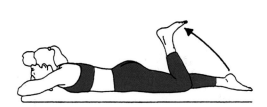

PRONE HIP EXTENSION

Lying on stomach as shown, tighten front thigh muscle and lift leg 8-10 inches from floor. Keeping knee locked and pelvis on the floor, slowly lower leg. Repeat 5 times on each side.

PRONE HAMSTRING CURLS

Lying on stomach as shown, legs straight, bend knee slowly, bringing heel toward buttocks as far as posibble. Repeat 5 times on each side.

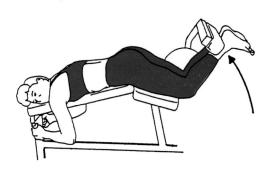

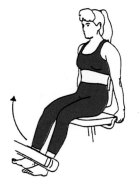

LEG CURL MACHINE

Adjust tension (weight) and leg curl apparatus. Lying face down on incline as shown, tighten leg muscles and bring heels toward buttocks. Progressively increase your weights.

LEG EXTENSION MACHINE

Adjust weight and seat height. Sitting upright as shown, tighten front thigh muscles and extend legs until knees are straight as possible, not locked. Progressively increase your weights.

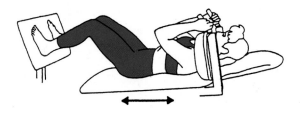

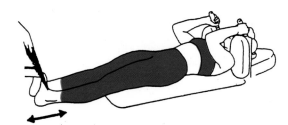

LEG PRESS MACHINE

Adjust weight and incline bench. Lying on bench as shown, tighten front thigh muscles and straighten legs. Keep back flat. Progressively increase your weight.

LEG PRESS MACHINE (FOR CALF STRENGTHENING)

Adjust weights and incline bench. Lying on bench as shown, tighten leg muscles and raising up on toes and back. Repeat 10 times.

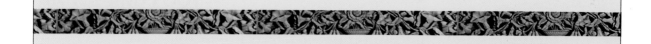

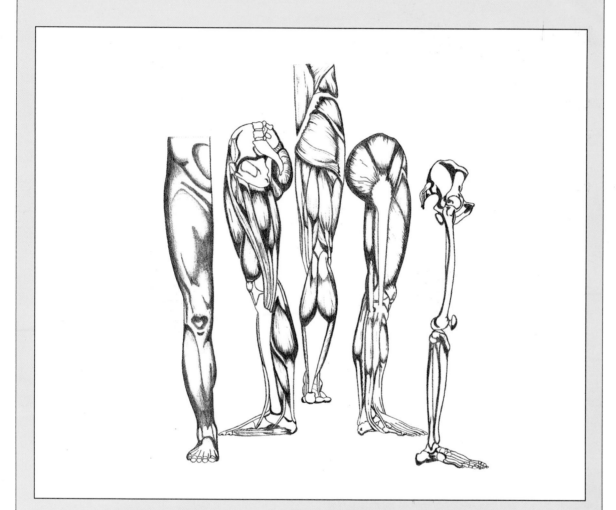

THE LOWER LEG
(ACHILLES, CALVES STRAIN & SHIN SPLINTS)

The Lower Leg

The back of the calf is comprised of two major muscles—one attached to the back of the thigh and one behind the knee. Both have lateral (outside) and medial (inside) heads, or starting points.

Close to the bottom of the calf muscle near the ankle, the Achilles tendon begins and inserts into the calcaneus (heel bone). This tendon, the largest in the body, needs to be as large as the muscle is strong. This tendon is often injured when stretched too quickly or repeatedly which causes an inflammation of the tendon or tendon trauma called Achilles tendinitis. The condition is characterized by sudden contractions of the calf muscle.

Other common causes of this condition are overuse and excessive pronation of the foot and ankle (the inward roll of the foot as it hits the ground) which causes the tendon to pull off-centered.

Calf muscle strains occur when too much pressure is exerted on the calf muscle.which causes the muscle and tendon to separate. These muscles lift the heel and propel the foot forward. This type of injury is more frequent with the onset of aging.

Sudden calf muscle contractions cause small rips or tears in the Achilles tendon. The tears and rips occur suddenly or accumulate over time. Occasionally, the Achilles tendon ruptures when the tendon is weak or lacking adequate blood supply.

Runners and joggers frequently complain of aching shins but the problem is usually pronating feet. Pronation of the foot is the inward roll as it strikes the ground when walking or running, sometimes called "flat feet." The foot, ankle and ligaments are loose and mobile. When weight is applied, the foot rolls to the inside, the ankle collapes inward, and the arch of the foot flattens out.

"Shin splints" are muscle pains near the shin bone caused by overuse or running on hard surfaces. While they usually occur in novice athletes, they can also plague the pro who has switched shoes, changed running surfaces, or has stepped up the paced of their workout.

True shin splint injury is rare. This term describes pain in the front of the inner side of the lower leg caused by strain or overuse resulting in the separation of muscle and tendon as well as inflammation of the muscle. Interruption of the blood supply or tibial stress fracture can also lead to shin splint conditions. Proper warm-up prior to exercise and a proper footwear can alleviate this problem.

Frequently shin pain is sometimes the result of "tibial stress syndrome." Excessive pronation causes an abnormal twist of the shin bone while the upper leg remains forward. The inward rotation combined with the shock and impact of running causes irritation and bone pain. Unrelieved bone stress can lead to fatigue and bone cracks. Excessive pronation can be reduced, however, with well-fitted shoes with an arch support.

The simplest way to prevent lower leg trauma is to maintain strong, flexible muscles. A regular exercise and stretching program helps to condition and to protect lower leg muscles, tendons and ligaments from strain or injury.

Achilles And Calves Strain
General Massage Areas

Maximum Pressure

35 LBS
25 LBS

Moderate Pressure

25 LBS
15 LBS

Minimum Pressure

15 LBS
5 LBS

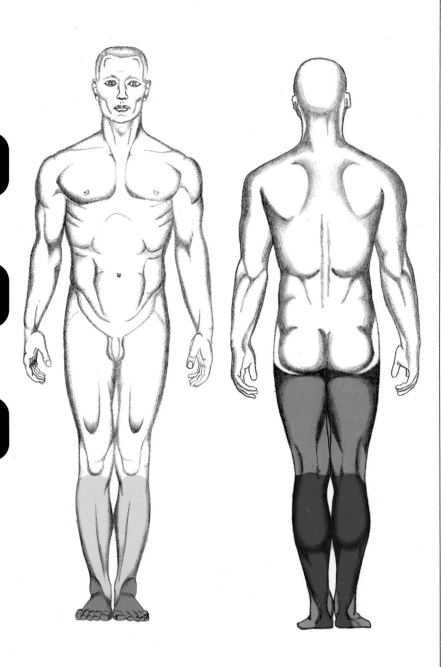

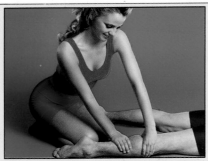

Before deep massage, knead the calf muscles with both hands.

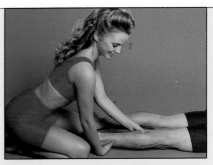

Use scorpion technique to nip down from the calf muscles to the achilles tendon.

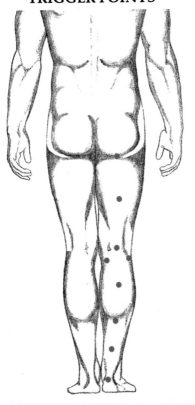

TRIGGER POINTS

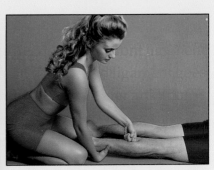

Use knuckle to manipulate trigger points around the calf.

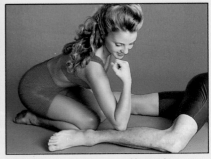

Use elbow technique on calf muscles.

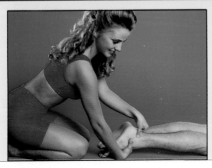

Use scorpion technique to relieve tightness of the achilles tendon.

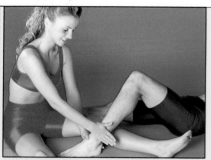

Apply palm technique for broad compression around the lower leg.

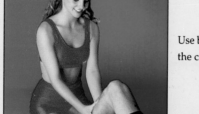

Use both hands to knead the calf.

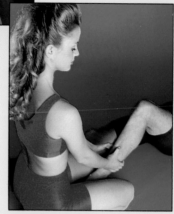

Use thumb technique to apply small circular pressure around the shin area.

TRIGGER POINTS

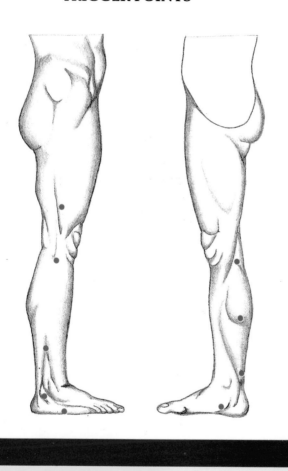

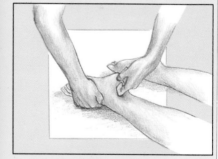

Use knuckle to make small circular motion on trigger point areas of the ankle.

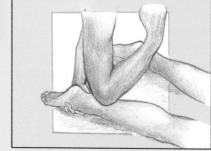

Use elbow to massage the archilles tendon.

Use elbow technique on large hamstring muscles, increase pressure gradually by applying body weight.

Shin Splints
General Massage Areas

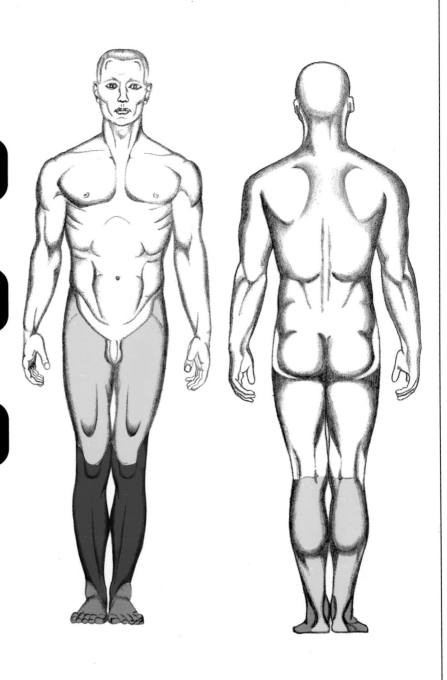

**Maximum
Pressure**

**35 LBS
25 LBS**

**Moderate
Pressure**

**25 LBS
15 LBS**

**Minimum
Pressure**

**15 LBS
5 LBS**

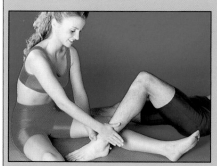

Apply palm technique for broad compression around the lower leg.

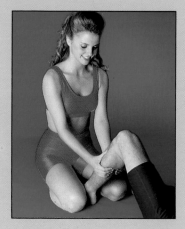

Use both hands to knead the calf.

TRIGGER POINTS

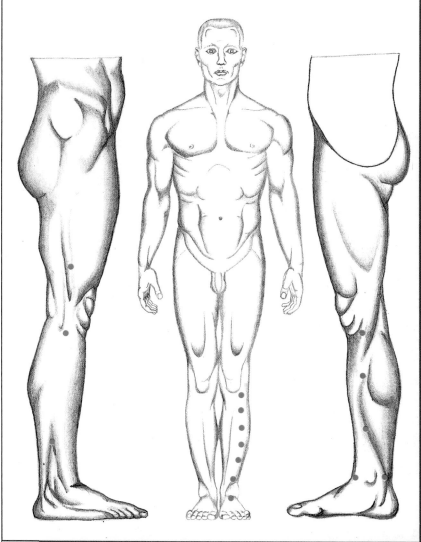

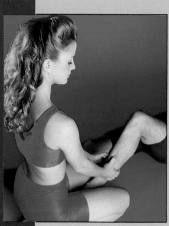

Use thumb technique to apply small circular pressure around the shin area.

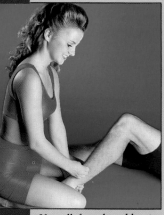

Use all four knuckles to apply circular motion around the shin area.

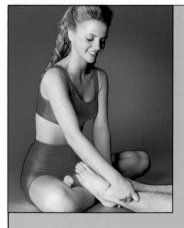

Apply knuckle technique on shin trigger points.

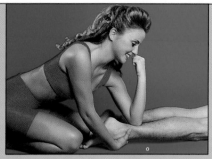

For deeper penetration, apply elbow technique to the lower leg muscles.

TRIGGER POINTS

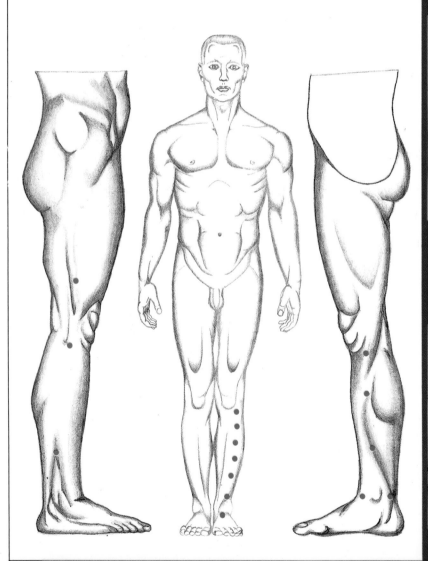

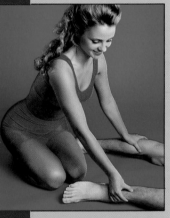

The thumb can be used to apply pressure to trigger points around the shin area.

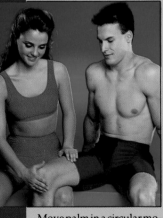

Move palm in a circular motion to relax tightness around the knee.

ACHILLES, CALVES STRAIN AND SHIN SPLINTS

S T R E T C H I N G

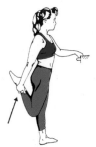

QUADRICEPS STRETCH

Standing at barre or counter, grasp ankle with hand as shown. Pull up slowly toward buttocks. Push pelvis forward to increase stretch. Hold 20 seconds. Repeat three times on each leg.

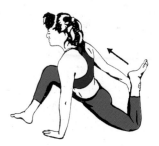

THE ATHLETIC QUAD STRETCH

Kneel on one knee, front leg at 90 degree angle as shown. With right hand grasp left foot, slowly lower front hip toward floor while gently pulling ankle toward buttocks. Hold 20 seconds. Repeat three times on each side.

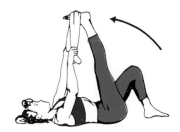

HAMSTRING STRETCH (WITH TOWEL)

Lying on floor, one knee bent as shown, loop towel around other foot. Tighten stomach muscles and raise leg up until slight tightness is felt. Keep knee joint locked and pull towards the head. Repeat three times with each leg.

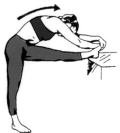

ATHLETIC HAMSTRING STRETCH (TABLE)

Stand erect with heel on counter or barre about hip height. Slowly roll upper body forward; place hands on foot, calf, or thigh. Hold stretch 20 seconds. Repeat three times each leg.

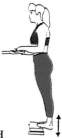

HEEL CORD STRETCH

With balls of feet on book or step, weight forward, hands grasping barre or counter, lower heels toward floor. Hold, then return to starting position. Do not bounce. Repeat 5 times.

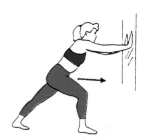

CALF STRETCH

Standing at wall with one foot back 3-4 feet from wall, opposite knee bent, lean against wall with hands. Lower hips until stretch is felt. Hold for 20 seconds, then repeat three times on each leg. Keep back leg straight, heels flat.

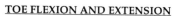

TOE FLEXION AND EXTENSION

Lying on back, legs straight, curl toes down then straighten and pull them towards body. Repeat ten times.

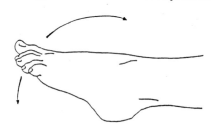

ANKLE PUMPS

Lying on back, legs straight, bend ankle to pull toes toward body. Then bend ankle to point toes away from body. Repeat ten times.

ACHILLES, CALVES STRAIN AND SHIN SPLINTS

S T R E N G T H E N I N G

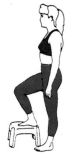

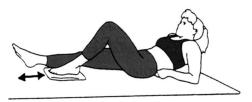

STEP UPS

Standing at side of 6-8" step, position foot on step as shown. Step up then down. Repeat twenty times.

HEEL SLIDE

Lying on floor as shown, flex knee and place a towel under the heel. Pull heel toward buttocks. Hold, then slide heel away to straighten leg. Repeat 3 times on each leg.

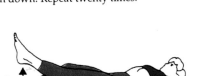

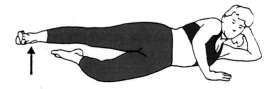

TERMINAL KNEE EXTENSION

Lying on back, place bolster under knees as shown. Lift foot up until leg is straight, knee supported by bolster. Hold, then slowly lower to starting position. Repeat 5 times on each side.

HIP ABDUCTION

Lying on side as shown, lower leg bent, top leg straight, raise top leg up 12-18 inches then slowly lower it. Hold for 10 seconds. Repeat 5 times on each side.

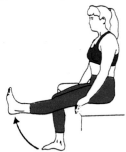

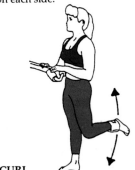

FULL ARC QUADS

Sitting upright in chair or on edge of table or bed as shown, extend leg until knee is straight. Hold for 10 seconds then lower leg to starting position. Repeat 5 times on each side.

HAMSTRING CURL

Standing up, hands holding barre or counter, cuff weight secured to ankle as shown, bend knee and raise heel toward buttocks. Slowly lower to starting position and repeat 10 times.

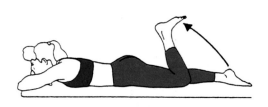

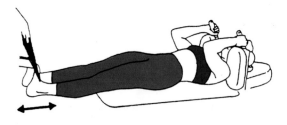

PRONE HAMSTRING CURLS

Lying on stomach as shown, legs straight, bend knee slowly, bringing heel toward buttocks as far as posibble. Repeat 5 times on each side.

LEG PRESS MACHINE (FOR CALF STRENGTHENING)

Adjust weights and incline bench. Lying on bench as shown, tighten leg muscles and raising up on toes and back. Repeat 10 times.

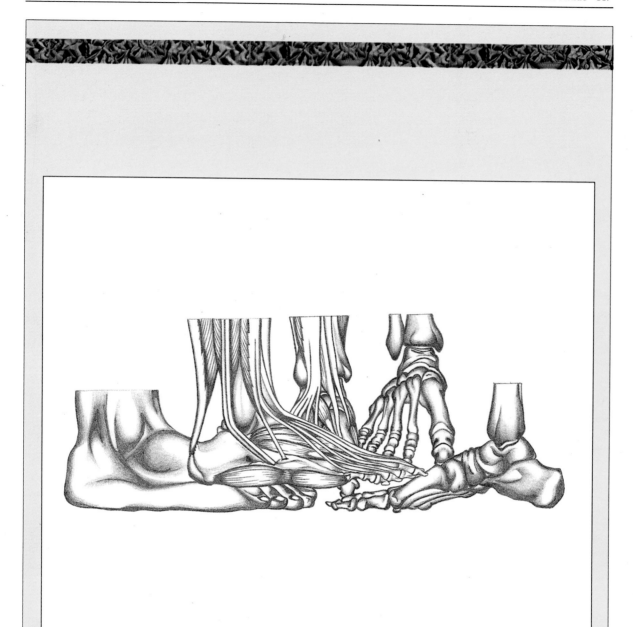

THE ANKLE

The Ankle

The ankle is one of the most primitive joints in the body and provides only up and down movement. Unable to rotate from side to side or inward and outward, the directional movement of the ankle is minimal and primarily stable.

Three major bones and two sets of ligaments comprise the ankle joint. The ankle bone fits into the space left by the two lower leg bones (tibia and fibula) and forms the top of the ankle joint. This space—or receptacle is called the mortice. The talus, or ankle bone, is covered with articular cartilage but is not attached with muscle or tendon.

The outer ankle bone is really the lower end of the smaller lower leg bone (fibula). The inner ankle bone is the lower end of the larger lower leg bone (tibia). The ends of both bones are covered with cartilage.

The deltoid ligament is on the inside of the ankle bone and attaches to the ankle itself. The outside ligament system is complex and runs in three directions. The front ligament extends from the lower leg bone down to the bones in the foot. The second ligament goes down the same area to the heel bone. The third ligament runs from the outer ankle knob directly to the bone of the foot. The outer ankle ligaments are generally weaker than the deltoid ligament, with 90 percent of all ankle sprains involved here.

Common ankle problems include ligament sprains, fractures, and Achilles tendonitis. When ankle ligaments are weak, the ankle bone can tip out if its mortice causing a sprain. Ligaments must be long and flexible for proper movement. Weak, short or tight ligaments can force ankle bones out of their sockets.

Ligament injuries and ankle sprains are one of the most common of all sports injuries and account for one-fifth of the visits to rehabilitation clinics. These sprains are divided into three types: outward sprain, which occurs when outside ligaments of the ankle are injured; inward sprain, where inside ligaments are injured; and forward sprain, which pulls the tendons in front of the ankle and tears the ankle capsule.

Ankle injuries usually result in swelling and tenderness and should be treated with ice. Untreated ligament injury can result in permanent instability. Ankle injuries should be completely rehabilitated with range of movement exercise and strength restored before resuming athletic training or activity.

Runners and joggers frequently complain of aching shins but the problem is usually excessive pronating of the feet. The foot, ankle and ligaments are loose and mobile. When weight is applied, the foot rolls to the inside, the ankle collapes inward, and the arch of the foot flattens out. The knees turn in, legs and hips are pulled out of line.

Conversely, a supinating foot has a rigid arch which fails to collapse when the foot strikes the ground, and the shock is sent up the outside of the leg rather than being absorbed by a flexible arch.

Both excessive pronation and supination can be corrected with proper athletic shoes fitted with an appropriate orthotic support.

The plantar fascia is the shock-absorbing pad that holds up the arch. Inflammation called plantar fasciitis causes dull aches along the arch. Running and jogging can cause overstretching or partial tearing of the plantar fascia which causes pain when exerting weight on the foot and pushing off for the next stride. Pulling on the plantar fascia where it attaches to the heel causes the heel bone to overgrow and form a painful "heel spur."

Even minor deviations from normal foot anatomy can cause injury if subjected to prolonged loading or shock. An abnormality of the foot can put stress up the leg to the back, increase muscle exertion, and accelerate overuse injuries.

In addition, runners frequently contribute to foot injuries by intensive training, running too far, running on hilly ground, changing surfaces, and inadequate recovery time.

Ankle And Foot Sprain
General Massage Areas

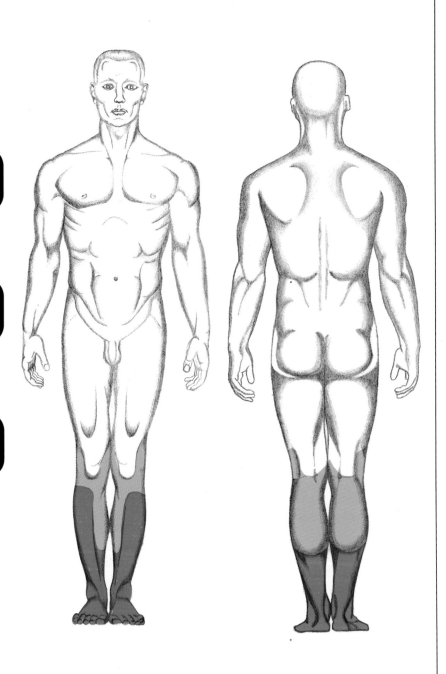

Maximum Pressure

35 LBS
25 LBS

Moderate Pressure

25 LBS
15 LBS

Minimum Pressure

15 LBS
5 LBS

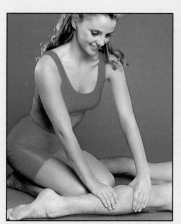

With both hands knead the calf muscles. Pressure should be alternated between the hands.

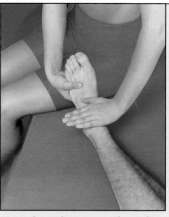

Use palm technique to relax tightness of the ankle area.

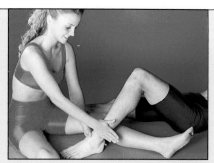

Apply palm technique for broad compression around the lower leg.

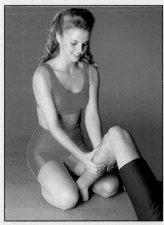

Use both hands to knead the calf.

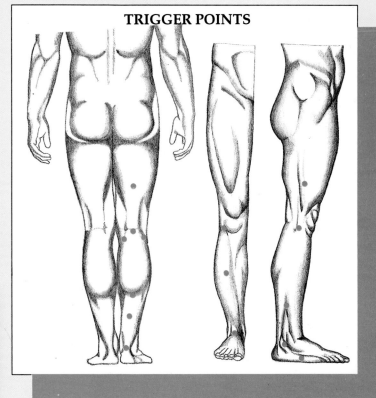

TRIGGER POINTS

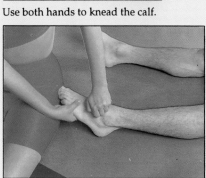

Use all four knuckles to massage ankle area.

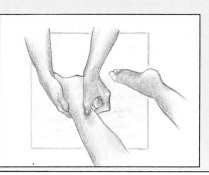

Use elbow to massage the archilles tendon.

Nip the achilles tendon, massage toward the calf using the scorpion technique.

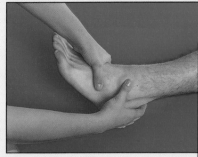

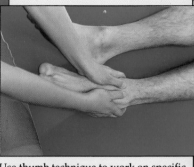

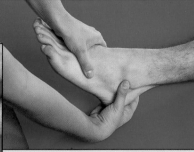

Use thumb technique to work in a circular motion around the stretched ankle area.

Use thumb technique to work on specific trigger points of the ankle.

Use thumb technique to gradually increase pressure around the ankle area.

TRIGGER POINTS

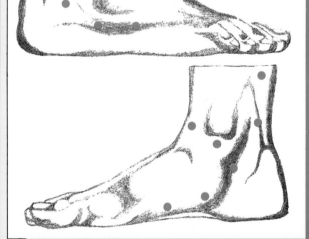

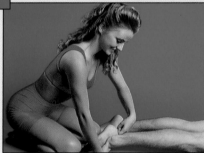

Use knuckle to make small circular motions on trigger point areas of the ankle.

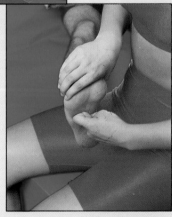

Use one hand to extent Receiver's toes. Use thumb technique on the sole of the foot.

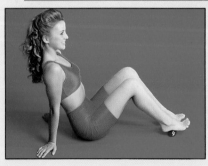

Use 3lbs. dumb bell weight place under both foot and press while rolling it. This will help release tighness of the plantar tendons under the foot.

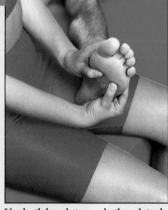

Use both hands to apply thumb technique to Receiver's foot and sole.

Use one hand to extend Receiver's toes. Use knuckle to make circular motion on the sole of the foot.

ANKLE AND FOOT
S T R E T C H I N G

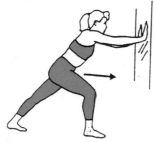

CALF STRETCH
Standing at wall with one foot back 3-4 feet from wall, opposite knee bent, lean against wall with hands. Lower hips until stretch is felt. Hold for 20 seconds, then repeat three times on each leg. Keep back leg straight, heels flat.

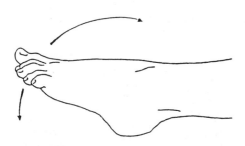

ANKLE PUMPS
Lying on back, legs straight, bend ankle to pull toes toward body. Then bend ankle to point toes away from body. Repeat ten times.

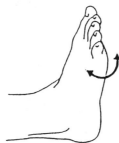

FOOT INVERSION AND EVERSION
Lying on back, legs straight, rotate ankle to turn foot inward so sole faces opposite foot. Then turn foot outward so sole faces away from opposite foot. Repeat ten times for each side.

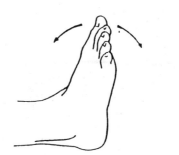

TOE FLEXION AND EXTENSION
Lying on back, leg straight, curl toes down then straighten and pull them towards body. Repeat ten times.

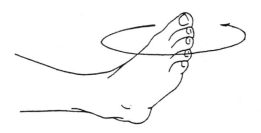

ANKLE CIRCLES
Lie on back with legs straight. Rotate feet around in circles as wide as possible. Circle ten times in one direction.

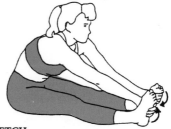

SHIN STRETCH
Sitting as shown, legs straight, rotate ankles to turn feet inward. Grab feet with hands at the arch and gently pull towards body. Hold stretch for 20 seconds. Relax and then repeat five times.

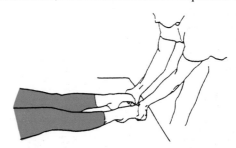

TOE STRETCH
Lying or sitting on floor or table, point toes against resistance of assistant. Apply gentle pressure. Hold stretch for 20 seconds. Repeat five times.

ANKLE AND FOOT
S T R E N G T H E N I N G

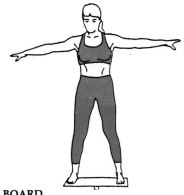

BALANCE BOARD
Standing on board as shown, arms relaxed and outstretched, balance body weight evenly until board is parallel to floor. Hold.

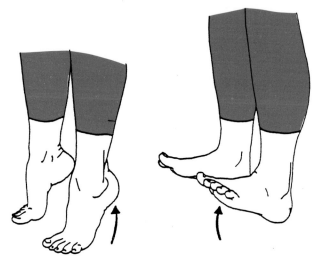

FOOT GRABBER
Sitting with foot on towel or cloth, curl toes under to pull and gather cloth under arch of foot. Release, then spread them out as far as possible. Repeat five times.

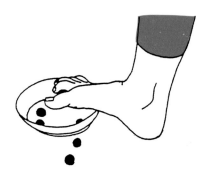

MARBLE PICK-UP
Sitting in chair, curl toes under to pick up marble with toes and drop it into dish. Repeat five times.

HEEL-TOE LIFT
Standing with feet slightly apart as shown, hands on hips for balance, lift toes off floor. Hold, then return toes to floor. Then lift heels off floor as high as possible. Repeat five times.

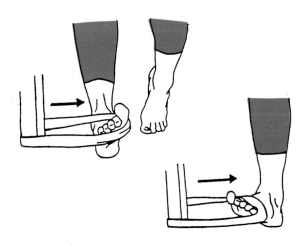

THERA-BAND EXERCISE
With thera-band attached to table leg and foot as shown, push foot outwards against the band. Repeat ten times on each leg.

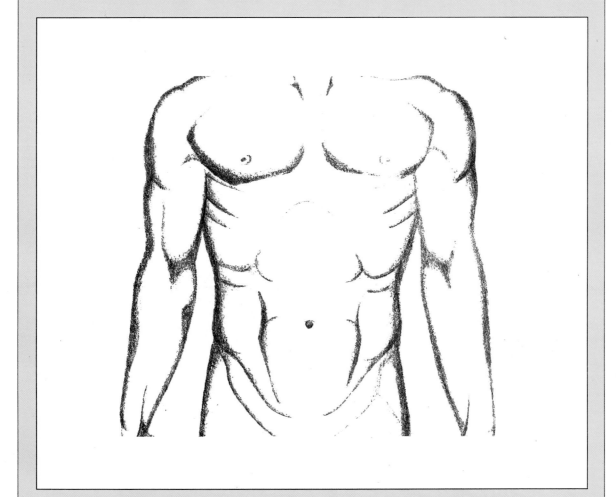

THE STOMACH

The Stomach

The stomach is often overlooked in massage. Eating disorders and poor exercise habits are just two of many reasons for stomach muscle and intestinal massage. Stomach massage improves circulation and muscle tone. The stomach is a complicated energy-producing machine that we depend on for digestion of food, nutrients, minerals, and vitamins. Since it is not protected by bones but by muscle, the stomach depends on exercise to prevent poor muscle structure. Massage promotes improved muscle structure and stimulates circulation.

Although an athlete's abdomen is usually not protected during play, abdominal injuries are not common in most athletic activities. An alert athlete can tense the abdominal muscles to prevent damaging blows to the spleen, liver and kidneys. Occasionally, however, an athlete will suffer a blow to the abdomen in contact events, or an over-zealous athlete will twist or stretch the abdominal muscle resulting in painful hematoma.

Malaysian midwives massaged the stomach before and after birth to improve muscle tone, to aid digestion, and to position the child. Ancient touch Masters performed stomach massage to alleviate fear and to compensate for the effects that fear has on the stomach and digestive system. The same ancient techniques help improve body functions and increase energy levels.

Stomach Cramps
General Massage Areas

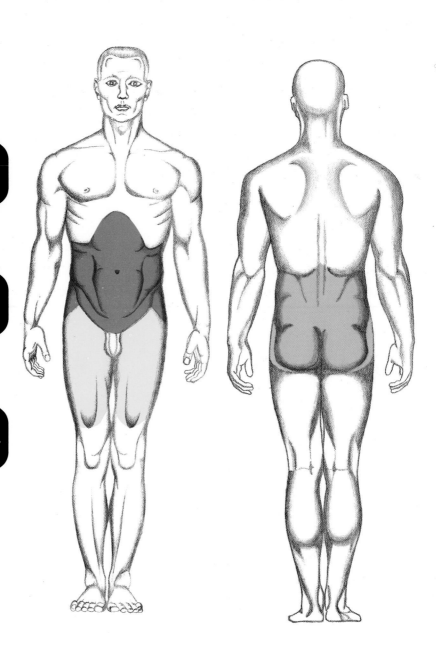

Maximum Pressure

35 LBS
25 LBS

Moderate Pressure

25 LBS
15 LBS

Minimum Pressure

15 LBS
5 LBS

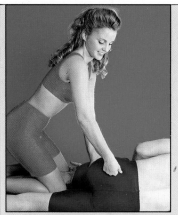

Use the thumb technique on trigger points around Receiver's sacro-iliac joint.

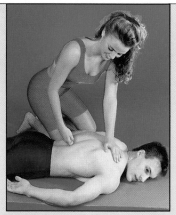

Use the knuckle technique to massage the back muscles in penetrating circular motions.

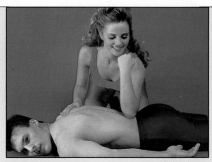

Use body weight to deeply massage the muscles of the lower back in a circular motion. Avoid the spine.

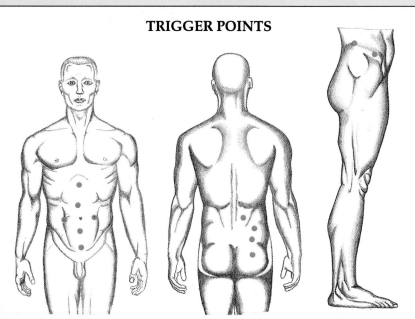

TRIGGER POINTS

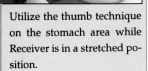

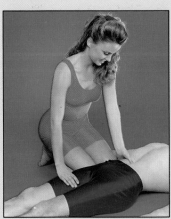

Utilize the thumb technique on the stomach area while Receiver is in a stretched position.

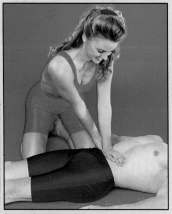

Move palm in a circular motion to relax the abdominal muscles. Increase depth gradually.

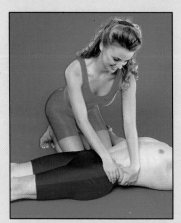

Use both hands to knead muscles around the waist.

Use the thumb to work under the ribs and on the trigger points of the stomach.

STOMACH

S T R E T C H I N G

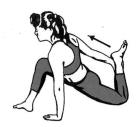

THE ATHLETIC QUAD STRETCH

Kneel on one knee, front leg at 90 degree angle as shown. With right hand grasp left foot, slowly lower front hip toward floor while gently pulling ankle toward buttocks. Hold 20 seconds. Repeat three times on each side.

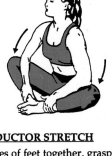

SITTING ADDUCTOR STRETCH

Sitting with soles of feet together, grasp ankles and press legs toward floor with elbows as shown. Hold stretch 20 seconds and release. If back is uncomfortable or tight, move feet away from body. Repeat three times.

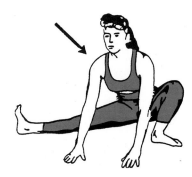

ATHLETIC GROIN STRETCH

Squat with one leg bent, one leg extended, arms forward as shown. Slowly lower hips toward floor. Hold stretch, then switch sides. Do not bounce. Use hands for stability. Repeat three times on each side.

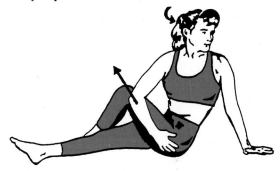

SPINAL TWIST

Sitting on floor with one leg crossed as shown, rotate upper body in direction of bent leg. Push against crossed leg until stretch is felt. Use free arm and elbow to press against leg to increase stretch. Hold stretch for 10 seconds. Repeat three times on each side.

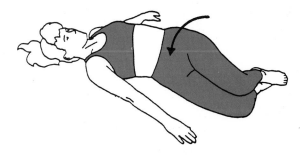

TRUNK ROLL

Lying on back with knees bent, feet flat, rotate hips and drop knees to one side. Keep shoulders and hand flat on the floor. Hold for 10 seconds. Return to starting position and repeat three times on each side.

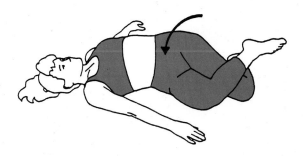

ATHLETIC TRUNK ROLL

Lie on back with knees bent. Cross one leg over the other, rotate hips, and push the lower knee to the floor. Hold 10 seconds, then repeat three times on each side. Keep shoulders and hands flat against the floor.

STOMACH
S T R E N G T H E N I N G

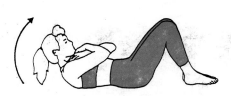

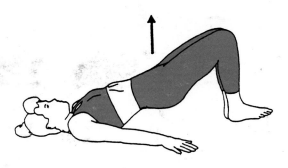

PARTIAL SIT-UP

Lying on back with knees bent, feet flat, arms crossed as shown, tuck chin toward chest and lift head and shoulders off floor. Using your stomach muscles "crunch" then return to floor. Do not hold breath. Repeat 10 times.

BRIDGING

Lying on back with knees bent, feet flat, tighten buttocks muscles and lift hips, back and buttocks off the floor. Hold 10 seconds. Repeat 10 times.

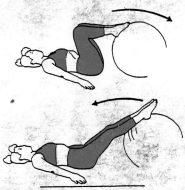

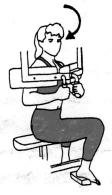

ATHLETIC LOWER ABDOMINAL

Lie on back, legs bent, feet on therapeutic ball as shown. Tighten stomach muscles and push ball away. When legs are straight, bring ball back. Press lower back into floor. Repeat 10 times.

ROTARY TORSO

Adjust weights, angle of torsion, and seat height. Press chest firmly against chest pad, grasp handles, and turn to one side. Exhale as you slowly turn to the other side. Control the machine's return; do not let the weights slam together on return. Do three sets of 10 repetitions. Progressively increase your weights.

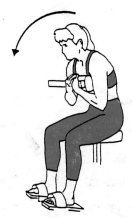

ABDOMINAL

Adjust weights, seat and leg height, and position arms as shown. Exhale as you lean forward, leading with the chest. Tighten stomach muscles to keep movements slow. Do not let weights slam together on return. Do three sets of 10 repetitions. Progressively increase your weights.